HASHIMOTO VEGETARIAN AUTOIMMUNE COOKBOOK

Your Roadmap to Reversing Symptoms, Improve Digestive Health, Beat Rheumatoid Arthritis, Systemic Lupus Erythematosus, and Graves' Disease

Daria Cross, MD

COPYRIGHT PAGE

The information in this book is not intended, under any circumstances, to replace or serve as a substitute for professional medical advice, diagnosis, or treatment. Any individual seeking advice regarding a medical condition or seeking treatment options should always consult with a qualified healthcare provider or physician. The author and publisher explicitly disclaim any responsibility for adverse effects or consequences arising from the utilization of the recipes or information presented in this cookbook.

Table of Contents

PART 1: INTRODUCTION TO HASHIMOTO'S THYROIDITIS

Hashimoto's disease is an autoimmune disorder that can lead to hypothyroidism, or an underactive thyroid. It is a chronic condition, meaning it lasts a lifetime.

The thyroid is a small, butterfly-shaped gland located at the front of your neck beneath the skin. It is part of the endocrine system and produces thyroid hormones.

The primary function of the thyroid is to regulate the speed of your metabolism, which is how your body converts food into energy. While metabolism is often associated with weight gain or loss, it actually influences every organ in your body, including the heart and brain.

In most cases of Hashimoto's disease, the thyroid is unable to produce sufficient thyroid hormone, leading to a slower metabolism and various symptoms.

The disease is named after Dr. Hakaru Hashimoto, who discovered it in 1912. It is also known as Hashimoto thyroiditis, chronic autoimmune thyroiditis, or lymphocytic thyroiditis.

Hashimoto's disease is quite common, affecting about 5% of people in the United States.

In countries where iodized salt and iodine-enriched foods are widely available, Hashimoto's disease is the leading cause of hypothyroidism. In other countries, iodine deficiency is the most common cause.

Thyroiditis refers to inflammation of the thyroid gland. Hashimoto's thyroiditis is the most prevalent form of this condition. As an autoimmune disease, it occurs when the body produces antibodies that attack thyroid cells, impairing the thyroid's ability to produce hormones. This often results in an underactive thyroid, or hypothyroidism, which requires medication to maintain normal thyroid hormone levels.

Factors that increase the likelihood of developing Hashimoto's thyroiditis include:

1. Gender: Women are about seven times more likely to develop the disease. It can sometimes start during pregnancy.

2. Age: Most cases occur between the ages of 40 and 60, though it can also affect younger individuals.

3. Heredity: The disease often runs in families, although no specific gene has been identified.

4. Autoimmune Diseases: Having other autoimmune disorders, such as rheumatoid arthritis or type 1 diabetes, increases the risk. Conversely, having Hashimoto's thyroiditis raises the risk for other autoimmune conditions.

Symptoms of Hashimoto's thyroiditis may include an enlarged thyroid gland (goiter), fatigue, weight gain, and muscle weakness. Treatment is not necessary if thyroid hormone levels are normal. However, medication can help if the thyroid is underactive.

Understanding Autoimmune Thyroid Disorders

Autoimmune thyroid disease results from a complex interplay of genetic and environmental factors, many of which are still unidentified. This disease arises when the mechanisms that regulate thyroid-reactive T and B cells fail. These autoreactive cells are likely present to some degree in everyone, but disease develops only when these cells escape immune tolerance. Both cell-mediated and humoral immune responses contribute to tissue damage in autoimmune hypothyroidism. In Graves' disease, the production of thyroid-stimulating antibodies (TSAbs) leads to hyperthyroidism. The thyroid interacts with the immune system in several ways during the development of autoimmunity, often worsening the disease. This multistep process suggests the potential for immunological treatments targeting the interactions between T cells and antigen-presenting cells (APCs) or immune-regulatory T cell subsets to restore normal tolerance and treat Graves' disease.

Hashimoto's disease, also known as Hashimoto's thyroiditis, chronic lymphocytic thyroiditis, or chronic autoimmune thyroiditis, is an autoimmune disorder that affects the thyroid gland. The thyroid, a butterfly-shaped gland located at the base of the neck below the Adam's apple, produces hormones that regulate many bodily functions.

In Hashimoto's disease, the immune system attacks the thyroid gland, leading to the destruction of hormone-producing cells and resulting in decreased hormone production, or hypothyroidism. Although anyone can develop Hashimoto's disease, it is most common among middle-aged women. The primary treatment involves thyroid hormone replacement therapy.

Thyroid disorders occur when the thyroid gland produces either too little or too much hormone, disrupting metabolism, body temperature, blood pressure, and heart rate, among other functions. These disorders can cause a variety of symptoms that often resemble those of other conditions, making accurate diagnosis crucial. To diagnose thyroid problems, healthcare providers typically perform a physical exam and order tests, such as thyroid blood tests and imaging tests like a thyroid scan or ultrasound, to determine the underlying issue.

Stages of Hashimoto

Hashimoto's thyroiditis is a prevalent autoimmune condition affecting the thyroid gland, leading to various symptoms and potential complications. It is the most common cause of hypothyroidism in the United States. Understanding the stages of Hashimoto's thyroiditis is crucial for effective management and treatment. Recognizing the signs and symptoms at each stage allows you to work closely with healthcare providers to optimize your care and improve your quality of life. Let's explore the stages of Hashimoto's thyroiditis to help you identify where you may be in your journey with this condition.

Stage 1: Increased Risk

In the first stage, the main characteristic is an increased risk of developing Hashimoto's thyroiditis or other autoimmune diseases due to genetic predisposition. During this stage, your thyroid functions normally, and your thyroid levels, including the thyroid peroxidase (TPO) antibody test used to diagnose Hashimoto's, are likely to be normal.

Although you are more susceptible to developing an autoimmune condition, it is not guaranteed that you will develop Hashimoto's or any other disease. Many people at this stage are unaware of their increased risk.

What to do?

- Monitor your symptoms.

- Get your thyroid tested regularly.
- Consider lifestyle changes to support thyroid health.
- Get your thyroid tested immediately if you become pregnant and exhibit any symptoms of hypothyroidism.

Stage 2: The Trigger Stage

In individuals with a genetic predisposition to autoimmune diseases like Hashimoto's, a specific trigger often marks the beginning of the disease.

Factors Influencing the Onset:

Gender: Hashimoto's is more common in women, often triggered by hormonal changes such as pregnancy or menopause. High levels of estrogen may also increase the risk.

Environmental Factors: Exposure to certain chemicals, pollutants, toxins, and infections can trigger an autoimmune response. Acute stress from events like surgery or injury, as well as chronic stress and poor sleep, can weaken the immune system and contribute to the onset.

Diet and Nutrient Deficiencies: Diets high in gluten, processed foods, sugar, and inflammatory fats can lead to inflammation and autoimmune responses. Deficiencies in nutrients such as iodine, selenium, and vitamin D can impact thyroid function and increase the risk.

Not everyone with a genetic predisposition will develop the condition in response to a trigger.

What to do?

- Monitor your symptoms.

- Get your thyroid tested regularly.

- Consider adopting the Autoimmune Protocol Diet.

- Eat a healthy, anti-inflammatory diet.

- Avoid environmental toxins.

- Ensure you get at least 7 hours of quality sleep nightly.

- Manage stress effectively.

- Consult your doctor if you plan to become pregnant.

- Get your thyroid tested immediately if you become pregnant.

- Consider the benefits of selenium, an essential trace mineral for regulatory and metabolic functions.

Stage 3: Activation and Infiltration

When a trigger activates Hashimoto's disease, the immune system begins producing antibodies that mistakenly attack the thyroid gland, causing inflammation.

Characteristics of This Stage:

Symptoms: Some people may experience fatigue, brain fog, mood changes, and weight gain, though others may have no symptoms.

Thyroid Function: The thyroid usually remains functional, producing sufficient hormones. TSH levels typically stay within the normal range, though TPO antibodies may be elevated. A thyroid ultrasound might show changes indicative of Hashimoto's.

Diagnosis: If antibodies are elevated or an ultrasound shows changes, you may be diagnosed with Hashimoto's. If Free T4 and Free T3 levels are normal, thyroid hormone replacement is not usually prescribed.

This stage can last several years and is an optimal time for diagnosis. Lifestyle changes can prevent progression to more severe hypothyroidism.

What to do?

- Monitor your symptoms.
- Get your thyroid tested regularly.
- Prioritize healthy lifestyle changes, including avoiding toxic exposures, ensuring good

sleep, proper nutrition, and stress management.

- Consult your doctor if you plan to become pregnant.
- Get your thyroid tested immediately if you become pregnant.

Stage 4: Subclinical Hypothyroidism

In this stage, the antibody attack on the thyroid gland intensifies, compromising the gland's ability to produce sufficient thyroid hormone. Thyroid tests may reveal a slightly elevated TSH level, typically within the reference range or at the upper limit. Even with a normal TSH level, Free T4 levels often fall at the low end of the range or below the cutoff.

Symptoms:

Some individuals may remain asymptomatic, while others begin to experience symptoms of hypothyroidism, including fatigue, brain fog, weight gain, hair loss, and sensitivity to cold. A goiter (thyroid swelling) may also develop.

Management:

If your TSH level is within the normal range, your doctor may recommend "expectant management," involving regular monitoring of thyroid hormone levels and prescribing medication only when thyroid values clearly fall outside the normal range.

Thyroid levels and symptoms may fluctuate during this stage due to increasing damage to the thyroid gland, causing erratic hormone release.

What to do?

- Take any prescribed thyroid medications regularly and correctly.
- Monitor your symptoms.
- Get your thyroid tested regularly.
- Prioritize healthy lifestyle changes, including avoiding toxic exposures, ensuring adequate sleep, proper nutrition, and stress management.
- Consult your doctor if you plan to become pregnant.
- Get your thyroid tested immediately if you become pregnant.

Stage 5: Full-Blown Hashimoto's/Hypothyroidism

Most Hashimoto's diagnoses occur at this stage. The thyroid gland can no longer produce enough thyroid hormone to meet the body's needs, resulting in elevated TSH levels and low Free T4 and Free T3 levels.

Symptoms:

Patients experience a full range of hypothyroidism symptoms, including severe fatigue, brain fog, weight gain, hair loss, cold intolerance, and more frequent and intense symptoms.

Management:

Thyroid hormone replacement medication is necessary to alleviate symptoms and restore thyroid hormone balance. However, this treatment does not prevent the immune system from continuing to attack the thyroid gland. Maintaining a healthy lifestyle can help reduce inflammation and slow the immune attack.

What to do?

- Take your thyroid medications regularly and correctly.
- Monitor your symptoms.
- Get your thyroid tested regularly.
- Prioritize healthy lifestyle changes, including avoiding toxic exposures, ensuring adequate sleep, proper nutrition, and stress management.

- Consult your doctor if you plan to become pregnant.

- Get your thyroid tested immediately if you become pregnant.

Stage 6: Thyroid Atrophy

The final stage of Hashimoto's disease is when the thyroid gland becomes severely damaged, leading to atrophy and an inability to produce thyroid hormone.

Not everyone with Hashimoto's reaches this stage. However, for those who do, lifelong thyroid hormone replacement medication becomes essential. While healthy lifestyle changes can support your treatment, replacing the missing thyroid hormone is crucial.

What to do?

- Take your thyroid medications regularly and correctly.
- Monitor your symptoms.
- Get your thyroid tested regularly.
- Prioritize healthy lifestyle changes, including avoiding toxic exposures, ensuring adequate sleep, proper nutrition, and stress management to help minimize autoimmunity.
- Consult your doctor if you plan to become pregnant.
- Get your thyroid tested immediately if you become pregnant.

Diagnosis and Symptoms

Hashimoto's thyroiditis is believed to stem from an immune defect influenced by environmental factors, although these factors aren't entirely understood.

Diagnosis relies on symptoms and laboratory findings. Elevated thyroid-stimulating hormone (TSH), reduced levels of free thyroxine (FT4), and increased anti-thyroid peroxidase (anti-TPO) antibodies in lab results are indicative of Hashimoto's thyroiditis. Some individuals also exhibit elevated TSH receptor-blocking antibodies

(TBII) and antithyroglobulin (anti-Tg) antibodies, both targeting the thyroid gland.

The destruction of the thyroid by the disease is intermittent. In its early stages, individuals may display symptoms and lab results resembling hyperthyroidism, or even have normal lab values. Consequently, detecting Hashimoto's thyroiditis can be challenging, and individuals may remain undiagnosed for months. Up to one-third of those treated for hypothyroidism receive inadequate or improper treatment.

While Hashimoto's thyroiditis affects both genders, women are 5–10 times more likely to receive a diagnosis. Risk increases with age, with most diagnoses occurring between 30 and 50 years old. For the general population, the peak age range for

Hashimoto's thyroiditis is typically between 45 and 65.

Treatment commonly involves synthetic or natural thyroid hormones. Synthetic options include levothyroxine (Synthroid) and liothyronine (Cytomel), whereas natural alternatives comprise Armour Thyroid and Nature Throid.

Symptoms

Because Hashimoto's thyroiditis impacts nearly every system in your body, it manifests with a range of symptoms. These can include:

- Weight gain
- Profound fatigue
- Difficulty concentrating
- Thinning, coarse hair

- Dry skin

- Slow or irregular heart rate

- Reduced muscle strength

- Shortness of breath

- Decreased ability to tolerate exercise

- Sensitivity to cold

- Elevated blood pressure

- Brittle nails

- Constipation

- Neck pain or tenderness in the thyroid area

- Feelings of depression and anxiety

- Menstrual irregularities

- Insomnia

- Changes in voice

Untreated or inadequately treated Hashimoto's thyroiditis can result in serious complications, including an elevated risk of heart disease, cognitive impairments, and in severe cases, even death.

PART 2: UNDERSTANDING HASHIMOTO'S THYROIDITIS AND DIET

Diet plays a crucial role in maintaining the health of the thyroid gland, which requires essential nutrients like iodine, selenium, and zinc to produce thyroid hormones. Insufficient intake of these nutrients can hamper hormone synthesis, potentially leading to thyroid dysfunction.

Hashimoto's thyroiditis is often fueled by inflammation. The immune system's attack on the thyroid gland triggers chronic inflammation, causing damage to the gland and impeding its hormone production. A diet rich in nutrients is suggested to alleviate symptoms and support thyroid health.

Key nutrients necessary for optimal thyroid function encompass iodine, selenium, zinc, vitamin D, omega-3 fatty acids, antioxidants, and fiber. Ensuring these nutrients are part of your daily diet may help maintain a balanced level of thyroid hormones.

While there isn't a one-size-fits-all diet for Hashimoto's, and no dietary regimen has been proven to cure the condition, thyroid hormone replacement medications can help manage symptoms. However, these medications do not address the underlying autoimmune process responsible for the thyroid attack.

The exact trigger for the autoimmune response damaging thyroid function remains unclear, but "leaky gut" or increased intestinal permeability might contribute. Gluten, found in wheat, barley, and rye, has drawn attention due to emerging research linking it to the production of a protein called zonulin in the intestine. Zonulin is believed to affect the tightness of intestinal cell connections, potentially allowing the absorption of substances triggering an immune response.

Individuals with Hashimoto's might also have celiac disease, another autoimmune condition that damages the small intestine. While celiac disease cannot be cured, it can be managed with a gluten-free diet. However, embarking on a gluten-free diet requires guidance from healthcare professionals, such as registered dietitian nutritionists, to devise an individualized nutrition plan. Poorly planned gluten-free diets may increase the risk of nutrient deficiencies, particularly in B vitamins, vitamin D, calcium, and iron.

Some individuals with Hashimoto's report symptom relief upon avoiding gluten. However, while an overwhelming majority in a survey felt better after adopting a gluten-free diet, a 2022 review found no evidence supporting the benefits of going gluten-free for Hashimoto's. It suggested that only individuals with celiac disease or gluten sensitivity should eliminate gluten from their diets.

Optimal Foods for Managing Hashimoto's Disease

Individuals with Hashimoto's often experiment with various diets, including vegan, paleo, grain-free, and dairy-free, hoping to alleviate symptoms. However, none of these diets have been scientifically proven to treat, cure, or reverse the condition. Instead, the most beneficial approach to eating with Hashimoto's focuses on mitigating inflammation while supplying nutrients that support overall health. Foods rich in antioxidants, found in whole fruits, lightly processed vegetables, and whole grains, are key contributors to reducing inflammation. Unsaturated fats and lean protein sources also play crucial roles in an anti-inflammatory diet plan.

1. **Diverse Fruits and Vegetables:** Incorporating a wide variety of fruits and vegetables daily ensures adequate intake of essential vitamins, minerals, and phytonutrients, which are natural plant compounds known for their protective properties. Many phytonutrients also act as antioxidants, combating inflammation.

2. **High-Fiber Foods**: Opt for fiber-rich foods like whole grains, legumes, beans, and vegetables to help regulate blood sugar levels, thereby reducing inflammation. Fiber also nourishes beneficial gut microbes that produce substances aiding in inflammation management. A well-balanced diet with sufficient fiber promotes weight control and supports heart health.

3. **Lean Proteins**: Sources of lean protein such as poultry, seafood, lean beef, eggs, tofu, beans, and legumes provide essential protein with minimal saturated fat content. Protein is vital for the production of immune system cells, crucial in managing autoimmune conditions like Hashimoto's.

4. **Healthy Fats:** Incorporate foods rich in monounsaturated and polyunsaturated fats, including omega-3 fatty acids, such as salmon, albacore tuna, nuts, flaxseeds, chia seeds, and avocados. These fats have anti-inflammatory properties, helping to reduce inflammation throughout the body.

Foods to Include for Thyroid Health

Your thyroid relies on iodine for proper functioning and to produce adequate thyroid hormone, as highlighted by the National Institutes of Health (NIH). Insufficient iodine intake can lead to hypothyroidism or a goiter, where the thyroid enlarges to compensate for the hormone deficiency, according to Medline Plus. While most Americans obtain sufficient iodine through iodized table salt, those on low-sodium or vegan diets may need to seek alternative sources.

Although various types of seaweed are rich in iodine, the iodine content can vary significantly. The iodine concentrations in different seaweed species range widely, with commercially available seaweeds containing anywhere from 16 mcg/g to

2,984 mcg/g, surpassing the recommended dietary allowance of 150 mcg for non-pregnant or non-lactating individuals, as per NIH guidelines.

While seaweed offers notable benefits, excessive consumption can pose risks to thyroid health. To enjoy the advantages without overdoing it, it is recommended to limit intake to one fresh seaweed salad per week, in addition to moderate sushi consumption, and avoiding seaweed teas and supplements.

1. Yogurt: Dairy products are a significant source of iodine, with an average of 85 mcg per cup, according to the NIH. However, iodine content in dairy can vary due to iodine supplements given to livestock and iodine-based cleaners used in the milking process. Plain, low-fat yogurt or Greek yogurt can contribute approximately 50% of the daily iodine intake, as suggested by the NIH.

2. Brazil Nuts: Rich in selenium, Brazil nuts aid in regulating thyroid hormones, potentially protecting against long-term thyroid issues such as Hashimoto's and Graves' disease, as indicated by a 2013 review in Clinical Endocrinology. Just one kernel contains between 68–91 micrograms of selenium. However, caution is advised not to exceed the upper limit of 400 micrograms per day, as excessive selenium intake can lead to adverse effects like "garlic breath," hair loss, nail discoloration, and even heart failure.

3. Dairy Products: Dairy, including milk and milk products, stands out as one of the richest sources of iodine, as stated by the NIH. However, plant-based milk alternatives like soy and almond beverages typically contain lower iodine levels.

Over the years, dairy consumption has seen a decline, according to data from the United States Department of Agriculture (USDA). Per capita fluid cow's milk intake has been decreasing steadily for more than 70 years, with a continued decline of approximately 1% per year during the 2000s and an accelerated average decline of 2.6% per year during the 2010s.

A single cup of low-fat milk can fulfill approximately one-third of your daily iodine requirements. Additionally, opting for milk fortified with vitamin D is advisable. A 2013 study in the *International Journal of Health Sciences* discovered a higher likelihood of vitamin D deficiency among individuals with hypothyroidism. Another noteworthy mention in the dairy category is cheese, particularly cheddar, which provides 12 micrograms of iodine and 7 IU of vitamin D per slice.

4. Poultry and Beef: Zinc plays a crucial role in thyroid function, as the body requires it to produce thyroid hormone. Insufficient zinc intake can lead to hypothyroidism, according to a 2013 study in the International Journal of Trichology. Interestingly, individuals with hypothyroidism may also become deficient in zinc, as thyroid hormones aid in zinc absorption. Such deficiency may result in severe alopecia, an autoimmune condition causing hair loss in clumps, as highlighted in a 2013 report in the same journal.

While most individuals in the US obtain sufficient zinc from their diet, those with poor dietary habits or gastrointestinal disorders hindering zinc absorption might be at risk of deficiency. Meats serve as a reliable source of zinc, with a 3-ounce serving of beef chuck roast providing 7 milligrams, a beef patty offering 3 milligrams, and 3 ounces of dark chicken meat containing 2.4 milligrams, according to the NIH.

5. Seafood: Fish serves as another excellent source of iodine, as highlighted by the American Thyroid Association, owing to the presence of iodine in soils and seawater. Research has shown that individuals residing in remote, mountainous areas devoid of access to the sea face an increased risk of goiters, as outlined in a 2014 study in BMC Public Health.

The absence of adequate nutrition is the most compelling evidence for thyroid problems. A 3-ounce serving of baked cod contains approximately 158 micrograms of iodine, meeting daily iodine requirements for non-pregnant or non-lactating individuals, as stated by the NIH. Even fish sticks provide a substantial amount of iodine, offering 58 micrograms in a 3-ounce serving.

6. Shellfish: Shellfish such as lobster and shrimp are generally rich in iodine. Just 3 ounces of shrimp, equivalent to approximately 4 or 5 pieces, contains around 10% of the recommended daily iodine intake, according to the NIH.

7. Eggs: A single large egg provides about 16% of the daily iodine requirement and 20% of the daily selenium requirement, making eggs a thyroid-friendly food, according to the NIH. Unless advised otherwise by your healthcare provider, consuming the entire egg is recommended, as much of the iodine and selenium content is concentrated in the yolk.

8. Berries: An optimal diet for thyroid health extends beyond iodine, selenium, and vitamin D. Antioxidant-rich foods, which combat cell damage, also contribute to thyroid well-being.

Berries, known for their high antioxidant content, are particularly beneficial. Black raspberries, a variant of raspberries with a deeper hue, stand out as one of the best choices, boasting high antioxidant levels, fiber, and relatively low natural sugar content, according to Johns Hopkins Medicine.

9. Cruciferous Vegetables: You might stumble upon claims online suggesting that cruciferous vegetables like broccoli, cauliflower, kale, and Brussels sprouts could potentially disrupt thyroid function. However, the reality is a bit more complex. While these veggies do contain compounds known as glucosinolates, which in high quantities might interfere with thyroid hormone production, consuming normal serving sizes is unlikely to cause harm to your thyroid.

A study published in Nutritional Reviews in 2016 revealed that the quantity and type of cruciferous vegetables consumed play a role. Eating typical servings of raw broccoli, Chinese cabbage, bok choy, or broccoli rabe is not expected to impair thyroid function. However, excessive intake, such as consuming more than 1 kg per day of raw Russian/Siberian kale, certain collards, and Brussels sprouts for several months, could reduce iodine uptake into the thyroid and impact thyroid hormone production.

10. Soy: The impact of soy on thyroid health has yielded inconsistent findings. Some concerns have been raised regarding soy's potential negative effects on thyroid function and hormone levels, as discussed in a 2019 meta-analysis published in Nature. However, after examining numerous studies, the authors concluded that soy supplementation did not influence thyroid hormones significantly.

As long as soy consumption remains within average amounts, there's little reason to fret over its impact on thyroid health.

Foods to Avoid or Limit

Some foods are typically advised against for thyroid health.

1. Gluten:

A 2021 review in Nutrients highlighted the frequent coexistence of celiac disease and autoimmune thyroid diseases like Hashimoto's thyroiditis and Graves' disease. This review suggested a significant thyroid-gut-axis, indicating that gut microorganisms not only impact the immune system and nutrient absorption but also thyroid function.

While it's uncertain whether a gluten-free diet alone can effectively treat thyroid disease, strict adherence to a gluten-free diet is crucial for managing symptoms if you've been diagnosed with celiac disease.

2. Processed Foods:

Considering increasing your iodine intake by indulging in salty, processed foods? Think twice. Manufacturers aren't obligated to use iodized salt in their products. According to the NIH, they rarely do. Consequently, you might be consuming excess sodium, risking high blood pressure and heart disease, without benefiting from iodine.

3. Fast Food:

Much like processed foods, fast-food establishments aren't mandated to incorporate iodized salt into their offerings. The American Thyroid Association advises against restaurant foods due to the lack of consistency in iodized salt usage. USDA analysis revealed that a fast-food hamburger patty contained 3.3 mcg of iodine per 100 g, whereas a non-fast-food ground beef patty contained 8 mcg of iodine per 100 g.

4. Goitrogens:

Goitrogens, found in cruciferous vegetables like cabbage and Brussels sprouts, as well as soy products, may disrupt thyroid hormone production. However, most individuals, including those with hypothyroidism, can safely enjoy moderate amounts of goitrogenic foods. Cooking these foods reduces their goitrogenic activity, rendering them safer for individuals with hypothyroidism.

Despite this, it's advisable for those with hypothyroidism to limit the intake of certain goitrogenic foods like cabbage, Russian kale, bok choy, Brussels sprouts, soy, and pearl millet. In general, it's prudent for individuals with hypothyroidism to moderate their consumption of goitrogenic foods.

Sample Meal Plan

Each person with hypothyroidism has unique health and dietary requirements. Caloric needs vary based on several factors, such as age, activity level, gender, height, and whether one aims to lose or gain weight. This basic meal plan offers insight into what a nutritious diet might entail for individuals managing hypothyroidism.

Monday

Breakfast: egg and spinach omelet served with half of an avocado and a bowl of berries

Lunch: a large green salad with chicken, beans, and pumpkin seeds

Dinner: stir-fried shrimp and vegetables served with brown rice

Tuesday

Breakfast: chia pudding with almond butter and berries

Lunch: grilled salmon salad

Dinner: fish baked with lemon, thyme, and black pepper served with roasted vegetables and a baked potato

Wednesday

Breakfast: egg and veggie muffins with a side of fruit

Lunch: Mediterranean quinoa salad with chickpeas, vegetables, and feta

Dinner: shrimp skewers and a salad

Thursday

Breakfast: spinach, chickpea, and sweet potato breakfast hash

Lunch: chicken salad with fresh veggies and fruit

Dinner: butternut squash and lentil curry

Friday

Breakfast: protein berry smoothie made with vanilla pea protein, natural peanut butter, and frozen mixed berries

Lunch: a large green salad with chicken, fresh vegetables, beans, and pumpkin seeds

Dinner: stuffed peppers

Saturday

Breakfast: egg, mushroom, and zucchini frittata

Lunch: Mediterranean tuna and quinoa salad

Dinner: brown rice pasta with chunky pasta sauce and chicken meatballs

Sunday

Breakfast: blueberry protein pancakes

Lunch: fish taco bowls

Dinner: sweet potato turkey chili

PART 3: TASTY, YUMMY RECIPES FOR HASHIMOTO'S VEGETARIAN DIET

RECIPES FOR BREAKFAST ON THE HASHIMOTO'S VEGETARIAN DIET

Zucchini Pappardelle with Pesto and Eggplant alla Norma

Ingredients

1 large eggplant

Salt

1 cup fresh mint leaves

1 1/2 cups fresh basil leaves

1/2 cup pine nuts, toasted

Pepper

4 cloves garlic

1 lemon, zested and juiced

1 lemon, zested and juiced

1/4 cup plus 3 tablespoons olive oil

1/2 cup freshly grated Parmigiano-Reggiano

3 firm small to medium zucchini

4 cups vegetable stock

1 teaspoon chile flakes

1 pint cherry tomatoes

1 cup crumbled ricotta salata

Instructions

Slice off half the eggplant skin and slice the eggplant into 1/2-inch thick discs. Then stack the discs and cut the eggplant into 1/2-inch-wide batons. Salt the eggplant and let it drain on a kitchen towel for 20 minutes.

Place the mint and 1 cup of the basil leaves with the toasted pine nuts in the bowl of a food processor. Season with salt and pepper and grate in 1 clove garlic. Add in the lemon zest and juice, then turn the processor on and stream in about 1/4 cup olive oil. Place the pesto in a large shallow bowl that you can serve the zucchini pasta from. Stir in the cheese.

Using a vegetable peeler and shaving the length of the zucchinis very thinly slice them into wide, pasta-like ribbons. If the zucchini are large and seedy, discard the seeds once you get to the center. Flip the zucchini over and peel until you reach seeds. If the zucchini are firm and small to medium in size you'll be able to use all of the vegetable.

Place the vegetable stock and 2 cups water in deep skillet.

Heat the remaining 3 tablespoons olive oil, 3 turns of the pan, in a large skillet and heat over medium-high heat. Add the eggplant to the hot oil and lightly brown, 6 to 7 minutes, tossing occasionally. Toss and combine with the chile flakes and remaining garlic. Add the tomatoes and cover the pan with a tight fitting lid. Shake the pan occasionally and cook until the tomatoes burst, 7 to 8 minutes more.

Meanwhile, heat the stock and water to low rolling boil, add the zucchini, and cook for 2 minutes. Use a spider or tongs to remove the zucchini to the pesto. Add 1 cup cooking liquids and toss to coat and combine, using additional cooking liquids if necessary. Top with extra cheese to serve.

Remove the lid from the eggplant and tear in the remaining 1/2 cup basil leaves. Toss to combine.

Serve the zucchini piled up on plate with the eggplant alongside, topping eggplant with crumbled ricotta salata.

Beans Bourguignon

Ingredients

1 ounce dried porcini mushrooms

1 1/2 cups boiling water

1/4 cup plus 1 tablespoon olive oil

1 pound cremini mushrooms, quartered

Kosher salt and freshly ground black pepper

3 small carrots (about 5 ounces), sliced 1/8 inch thick

1 medium onion (about 10 ounces), chopped

2 tablespoons tomato paste

2 tablespoons fresh thyme leaves, chopped

1 teaspoon fresh oregano leaves, chopped

2 cloves garlic, thinly sliced

1 1/2 cups vegan dry red wine, such as cabernet sauvignon

8 ounces frozen pearl onions (about 2 cups)

Two 15-ounce cans cannellini beans, drained and rinsed

1 cup fresh flat-leaf parsley leaves, finely chopped, plus more for garnish, optional

12 ounces cavatappi pasta

Instructions

Place the porcini mushrooms in a medium heat-safe bowl. Pour the boiling water over top and let the porcini soak until the liquid is a very dark brown, about 20 minutes. Strain the liquid into a small liquid measuring cup (you should have about 3/4 cup), then chop the porcini and set aside.

Meanwhile, heat 2 tablespoons of the olive oil in a large heavy-bottomed pot over medium-high heat until shimmering. Add the cremini mushrooms, 1 teaspoon salt and a generous amount of black pepper and stir so the cremini are in an even layer. Let the cremini cook, untouched, until starting to caramelize, about 3 minutes. Stir the cremini a few times and then continue to cook, untouched, until golden brown, about 3 minutes more. Transfer to a medium bowl with a slotted spoon and return the pot to the burner.

Add another 2 tablespoons of the olive oil to the pot along with the carrots, onion, 1/2 teaspoon salt and a few grinds of black pepper. Cook, stirring occasionally, until the vegetables are softened, 4 to

5 minutes. Stir in the tomato paste, thyme, oregano, garlic and reserved porcini and cook, stirring frequently, until the tomato paste is toasted and turns a deep maroon color, 2 to 3 minutes.

Stir in the wine, bring to a simmer and cook until reduced by half, 3 to 4 minutes. Fold in the pearl onions, cannellini, cremini, reserved porcini water, 1 teaspoon salt and a few grinds of black pepper and bring to a simmer. Cook, stirring occasionally, until the sauce is thick enough to coat the back of the spoon and the mushrooms are very soft, 8 to 10 minutes. Fold in 1/2 cup of the parsley.

Meanwhile, bring a large pot of salted water to a boil. Cook the pasta until al dente according to package directions. Drain the pasta and add it back to the pot. Stir in the remaining 1 tablespoon olive oil and 1/2 cup parsley, 1 teaspoon salt and a few grinds of black pepper. Serve the beans bourguignon on top of the herbed pasta and garnish with more parsley if desired.

Vegan Mac N "Cheeze"

Ingredients

Breadcrumb Topping:

1 slice gluten-free bread

1 teaspoon olive oil

1/2 teaspoon garlic powder

1/4 teaspoon paprika

1/4 teaspoon kosher salt

Pasta:

One 8-ounce box dried chickpea pasta or your favorite pasta

1 tablespoon olive oil

1/2 onion, diced

1 carrot, sliced

1 stalk celery, roughly chopped

2 cups peeled and cubed butternut squash

1/2 cup raw cashews

1 1/2 teaspoons fine sea salt

2 tablespoons nutritional yeast

1/4 teaspoon garlic powder

Torn fresh parsley leaves, for serving

Instructions

Bring a large pot of water to a boil.

Heat the olive oil in a large saucepan over medium heat. Add the diced onion and cook until softened, 1 to 2 minutes.

Add the celery and carrots and cook until the vegetables have softened, 1 to 2 minutes. Add the butternut squash and cook until slightly browned, 6 to 8 minutes. Add just enough water (about 2 cups) to barely cover the vegetables. Add the cashews and 1 teaspoon salt, bring to a boil and cook until the vegetables are tender when pierced with a fork, about 10 minutes, but cooking time will vary slightly, depending on the size of the vegetables.

For the pasta:

Salt the water and cook the pasta to al dente according to package instructions. Drain and set aside.

For the breadcrumb topping: Roughly chop the bread and pulse in a food processor until the bread resembles coarse crumbs. Heat the oil in a small skillet over medium-high heat. Add the breadcrumbs, garlic powder, paprika and salt and toss to combine. Cook, tossing regularly, until golden and crispy, 3 to 5 minutes.

Transfer the vegetable-cashew mixture to a blender along with the remaining cooking liquid. Blend until smooth, then add the nutritional yeast, garlic powder and the remaining 1/2 teaspoon salt. Blend until smooth, then taste and adjust the seasoning to taste.

Pour the creamy sauce over the cooked pasta and toss to combine.

Sprinkle with crispy breadcrumbs and parsley and serve.

Vegan Tostadas

Ingredients

1 cup raw walnuts

1 cup canned black beans, rinsed and drained

2 tablespoons extra-virgin olive oil

1/2 medium yellow onion, diced

1 garlic clove, minced

1 cup canned diced tomatoes with juices

1 tablespoon ground cumin

1 tablespoon dried oregano

1/2 teaspoon cayenne pepper (optional)

Kosher salt and freshly ground black pepper

6 organic corn tortillas

1 cup vegan shredded cheese (optional)

Optional Toppings:

Pepitas

Canned sweet yellow corn, drained

Diced red bell pepper

Sliced avocado

Shredded lettuce

Vegan cheese sauce, warmed (if not using shredded cheese)

Preheat the oven to 400 degrees F.

Instructions

Place the walnuts in a large skillet and cook over high heat, stirring occasionally, until toasted, about 3 minutes. Transfer the nuts to a food processor and reserve the skillet. Add the beans to the food processor and pulse with the nuts until the mixture is fully incorporated but not mushy. Set aside.

Heat 1 tablespoon of the oil in the same skillet over medium heat. Add the onions and garlic and cook, stirring, until the onions are softened, 2 to 3 minutes.

Add the bean mixture, tomatoes, cumin, oregano and cayenne, and stir to incorporate. Cook until the mixture is heated through, about 5 minutes.

Meanwhile, brush both sides of each of the corn tortillas with the remaining oil. Place on a baking sheet and bake until crispy, flipping halfway through, about 6 minutes total.

Remove the tostadas from the oven and top with the bean mixture, then the shredded cheese. Bake until the cheese is melted, about 5 minutes.

Add your desired toppings and enjoy!

Drunken Noodles

Ingredients

Sauce:

5 tablespoons (75 ml) Chinese sweet soy sauce

3 tablespoons (45 ml) Chinese vegetarian oyster sauce

3 tablespoons (45 ml) Thai soybean sauce (the label will say, "seasoning sauce")

2 tablespoons (30 g) vegan sugar

2 teaspoons (10 ml) Sriracha

2 teaspoons (10 g) minced garlic

6 to 8 Thai basil leaves, thinly sliced

Drunken Noodles:

3 tablespoons (45 ml) canola or peanut oil

2 to 3 garlic cloves, minced

1 to 2 serrano chiles, thinly sliced

5 ounces (145 g) extra-firm tofu in water, drained
and diced

1/2 medium white onion, sliced

3 to 4 cups (675 to 910 g) fresh rice noodles,
separated

1 cup (240 g) loosely packed Thai basil leaves

1/2 cup (120 g) grape tomatoes, halved

Instructions

For the sauce:

Combine the sauce ingredients in a small bowl, stir
together, and then set aside.

For the noodles:

Heat the oil in a medium sauté pan over medium-high heat. At the first wisp of white smoke, cook the garlic and serrano, stirring, until the garlic is light brown, about 1 minute. Add the tofu and onions, stirring constantly, until the tofu starts to brown, 1 to 2 minutes. Add the noodles and cook, tossing, until the noodles are soft and slightly browned on the edges, about 2 minutes. Add the sauce, basil, and tomatoes. Cook, tossing to combine, until the noodles completely absorb the sauce, 3 to 5 minutes.

NOTE: Check the label to be sure your soybean sauce is vegan.

Stuffed Peppers

Ingredients

Stuffed Peppers:

6 medium sweet bell peppers

2 tablespoons vegetable oil

2 cloves garlic, minced

1 medium onion, diced

Two 14.5-ounce cans chopped tomatoes

Kosher salt and freshly ground black pepper

One 14.5-ounce can corn kernels, rinsed

One 14.5-ounce can black beans, rinsed

3 cups baby spinach

1 cup cooked quinoa

2 teaspoons chili powder

1 teaspoon ground cumin

1 tablespoon chopped fresh cilantro

Vegan Cilantro-Lime Cream:

1/2 cup vegan sour cream or vegan cream cheese

1 teaspoon lime zest plus 1 tablespoon lime juice

2 tablespoons chopped fresh cilantro

Kosher salt

Instructions

For the stuffed peppers:

Preheat the oven to 350 degrees F.

Cut off the bell pepper tops, up to about 1/2 inch; discard the stems. Cut the tops into small dice and reserve. Discard the seeds and white membranes from the insides of the peppers. If a pepper doesn't stand upright, trim the bottom until level.

Add the oil to a large sauté pan over medium heat. Add the garlic, onion and diced bell pepper and cook until the onion is translucent, about 5 minutes. Mix in the tomatoes and season with salt and pepper.

Transfer 1 1/2 cups of the tomato mixture to an 8-by-11-inch baking dish and use a spatula or spoon to spread over the bottom of the dish. Set aside.

Add the corn, black beans, spinach, quinoa, chili powder and cumin to the remaining tomato mixture in the sauté pan. Cook on low heat until the spinach is fully wilted, 3 to 4 minutes. Remove from the heat and add the cilantro. Season with salt and pepper and let cool for 5 minutes.

Spoon the quinoa mixture into the cavity of each pepper, packing the mixture in. Arrange the peppers side by side in the baking dish and cover with foil. Bake until the peppers are tender, about 45 minutes.

For the vegan cilantro-lime cream:

Whisk together the sour cream, lime zest and juice and cilantro in a small mixing bowl until smooth and combined. Season with salt.

Top the peppers with the cream immediately before serving.

Vegan Tuna Noodle Casserole

Ingredients

Kosher salt and freshly ground black pepper

1 pound medium pasta shells

1/4 cup olive oil

1 pound cremini mushrooms, thinly sliced

1 tablespoon fresh thyme leaves, chopped

2 cloves garlic, minced

1 large onion, chopped

2 cups vegetable stock

1/4 cup all-purpose flour

1 cup cashew milk

1/3 cup vegan cream cheese

2 tablespoons vegan soy sauce

One 15-ounce can garbanzo beans, drained and rinsed

One 12-ounce block extra-firm tofu, pressed and crumbled

1 cup frozen peas

30 vegan butter crackers, such as Ritz (from 1 sleeve), crushed (about 1 1/2 cups)

1 cup fresh flat-leaf parsley, chopped

Hot sauce, for serving, optional

Instructions

Preheat the oven to 350 degrees F.

Bring a large pot of salted water to a boil and cook the pasta until not quite al dente, 6 to 7 minutes. Drain and add back into the pot, then toss with 1 tablespoon of the olive oil; set aside.

Meanwhile, heat the remaining 3 tablespoons olive oil in a large skillet over medium-high heat. Add the mushrooms, 1 1/2 teaspoons salt and a generous amount of pepper and cook, stirring occasionally, until almost all of the excess moisture has cooked off and the mushrooms start to turn golden brown,

6 to 7 minutes. Add the thyme, garlic and onions and continue to cook, stirring, until the onions begin to soften, about 2 minutes.

Pour 1/4 cup of the vegetable stock into the skillet and use a wooden spoon to scrape up any browned bits from the bottom. Simmer until the broth is reduced completely, about 3 minutes. Sprinkle the flour over the vegetables and cook, stirring, until completely absorbed. Add the cashew milk, remaining 1 3/4 cups vegetable stock, 1 teaspoon salt and a generous amount of pepper and cook, stirring, until thickened, 3 to 4 minutes. Stir in the cream cheese and soy sauce until smooth. Taste and adjust the seasoning with salt and pepper.

Add the garbanzo beans, tofu, peas and the mushroom sauce to the pot with the pasta and fold until well combined. Transfer the mixture to a 9-by-13-inch baking dish and sprinkle the crushed crackers on top. Bake until the casserole is warmed through and bubbling around the edges and the crackers start to turn golden brown, about 20 minutes. Let sit for 5 minutes, then sprinkle with the parsley. Serve with hot sauce on the side, if desired.

Mushroom Mapo Tofu

Ingredients

2 ounces dried shiitake mushrooms, washed (or 10 ounces creminis or fresh shiitake mushrooms)

1 tablespoon cornstarch

4 tablespoons vegetable oil

1 tablespoon minced ginger

1 tablespoon douchi (fermented black beans), chopped

1 tablespoon plus 1 1/2 teaspoons doubanjiang (spicy bean paste)

1 teaspoon Sichuan peppercorn powder, plus more for garnish

3 cloves garlic, minced

1 dried chile, such as Thai bird chile, chopped, optional

One 16-ounce block soft tofu, cut into 1-inch cubes

1 tablespoon soy sauce

1/2 teaspoon sugar

2 scallions, thinly sliced on a diagonal

1/2 teaspoon toasted sesame oil

Instructions

Put 2 cups cold water and the dried shiitake mushrooms in a small pot and bring to a boil. Turn off the heat and let sit to rehydrate for 30 minutes.

Squeeze excess water from the mushrooms, cut off and discard the stems and finely chop the mushrooms. Measure the mushroom-soaking liquid and add enough cold water to come to 1 1/2 cups.

Mix the cornstarch and 2 tablespoons cold water in a small bowl until combined; set aside.

Heat 2 tablespoons of the vegetable oil in a wok or large high-sided skillet over medium-high heat until it starts to smoke. Add the shiitakes and cook until browned, about 4 minutes. Lower the heat to medium, add the remaining 2 tablespoons vegetable oil, the ginger, douchi, doubanjiang, Sichuan peppercorn powder, garlic and dried chile, if using, and cook until everything is bright red, about 1 minute.

Add the mushroom-soaking liquid to the wok, scraping any brown bits off the bottom. Gently stir in the tofu and bring to a boil. Add the soy sauce and sugar, then stir in the cornstarch slurry and half of the scallions. Bring to a simmer and simmer until the sauce is glossy, about 1 minute.

Transfer to a serving dish, sprinkle with the remaining scallions and more Sichuan peppercorn powder if desired and drizzle the toasted sesame oil on top.

BBQ Spaghetti Squash Sliders

Ingredients

1 small spaghetti squash (about 3 pounds)

Kosher salt

3/4 cup of your favorite barbecue sauce

3 tablespoons pure maple syrup

2 tablespoons tomato paste

2/3 cup plus 2 tablespoons apple cider vinegar

2 teaspoons mayonnaise

1/4 small head red cabbage, finely chopped

1/4 small red onion, finely chopped

24 mini slider buns

1 English cucumber, cut into 1/4-inch-thick slices

Instructions

Preheat the oven to 350 degree F; line a baking sheet with foil.

Halve the squash lengthwise and scoop out the seeds. Season the flesh generously with salt and brush with 1/4 cup of the barbecue sauce. Arrange flesh-side down on the prepared baking sheet and roast until tender and the squash strands are easily separated with a fork, 45 minutes to 1 hour. Let cool for a few minutes on the baking sheet.

Meanwhile, whisk together the maple syrup, tomato paste, 2/3 cup of the vinegar, remaining 1/2 cup barbecue sauce, a pinch of salt and 1 cup water in a small saucepan. Bring to a boil, then reduce to a simmer and cook until thickened, 15 to 20 minutes. Keep warm.

Mix together the mayonnaise, cabbage, onion and remaining 2 tablespoons vinegar in a medium bowl. Season with salt.

Use a fork to separate the squash strands (keep them in the skins). Divide 1 1/4 cups of the sauce between the 2 halves and mix until the squash strands are coated. Season with salt.

Slice the buns open about three-quarters of the way. Divide the cucumber slices among the buns. Fill each with a generous amount of the squash and top with some slaw. Serve with extra sauce on the side.

Vegetarian Enchiladas

Ingredients

Sauce:

2 tablespoons vegetable oil

1/2 small onion, diced

2 cloves garlic, chopped

2 teaspoons ancho chile powder

1 teaspoon ground cumin

Large pinch cayenne pepper

One 15-ounce can tomato puree

Kosher salt

Filling and Topping:

One 10-ounce package frozen chopped spinach, thawed

One 15-ounce can pinto beans, strained and rinsed

4 ounces shredded Cheddar (about 1 1/2 cups)

4 ounces shredded pepper Jack cheese (about 1 1/2 cups)

1/2 cup sour cream

3 scallions, sliced

Kosher salt

Twelve 6-inch corn or flour tortillas

Juice of 1/2 a lime

Instructions

Special equipment: a 9-by-13-inch baking dish

Preheat the oven to 350 degrees F.

For the sauce:

Heat the oil in a large skillet over medium heat. Add the onions, and cook, stirring frequently, until soft and translucent, about 5 minutes. Add the garlic, chile powder, cumin and cayenne, and continue to cook, stirring, until the spices are toasted, about 1 minute. Add 2 cups water, the tomato puree and 1/2 teaspoon salt, and bring to a simmer. Continue cooking until the sauce reduces and thickens slightly (it should be looser and thinner than marinara sauce), 15 to 20 minutes. Set aside to cool slightly.

For the filling:

Squeeze all the excess moisture out of the spinach. Put it into a large bowl with the pinto beans, and squeeze with your hands to combine and smash up the beans a little. Add half of both the Cheddar and the pepper Jack, half of both the sour cream and the scallions and 1 1/4 teaspoons salt, and stir to combine.

Spread about 1/2 cup of the tomato sauce in the bottom of a 9-by-13-inch baking dish. Lay the tortillas out on a work surface, and spread 1 side of each with about 1 teaspoon of tomato sauce. Put about 1/4 cup of the filling across the middle of each tortilla. Roll each up, then shingle them in 2 even rows in the baking dish. Pour the remaining sauce over the top of the rolled tortillas, and sprinkle with the remaining cheeses. Cover the baking dish loosely with foil, and bake until the cheeses are melted and the filling is hot, about 30 minutes. Uncover, and continue baking to heat completely through, about 10 minutes more.

For the topping:

Whisk together the remaining sour cream, the lime juice and a pinch of salt in a small bowl. Drizzle the mixture over the baked enchiladas, and sprinkle with the remaining scallions.

Vegan Picadillo

Ingredients

2 tablespoons olive oil

1/2 yellow onion, diced

1/2 green bell pepper, diced

Kosher salt and freshly ground black pepper

3 cloves garlic, minced

2 teaspoons ground cumin

1 teaspoon dried oregano

24 ounces plant-based ground meat

1 tablespoon tomato paste

1/2 cup vegan-friendly vino seco or sherry cooking
wine

One 15-ounce can tomato sauce

1 bay leaf

1/4 cup pimiento-stuffed olives, halved crosswise

Juice of 1 lime

Cooked white rice, for serving

Instructions

Heat a medium skillet over medium-high heat. Add the oil, onion and bell pepper. Season with 1 teaspoon salt and a few cracks of black pepper. Cook, stirring occasionally, until the vegetables soften, 4 to 5 minutes. Add the garlic, cumin and oregano and stir until fragrant, about 30 seconds. Add the plant-based meat and cook until no longer pink, 5 to 6 minutes.

Stir in the tomato paste. Add the vino seco and scrape up any browned bits from the bottom of the skillet with a wooden spoon. Stir in 1 cup water, the tomato sauce and bay leaf. Simmer, stirring occasionally, until the tomato sauce thickens and turns a deep red color, 10 to 15 minutes.

Stir in the olives and lime juice. Discard the bay leaf. Serve the picadillo with the rice.

Baked Ziti with Mushrooms

Ingredients

9 tablespoons extra-virgin olive oil, plus more for drizzling

6 cloves garlic, thinly sliced

1 teaspoon dried oregano

Pinch of red pepper flakes

2 28-ounce cans whole peeled San Marzano tomatoes, crushed by hand

Kosher salt and freshly ground pepper

1 pound ziti

1 pound cremini mushrooms, sliced

1 cup vegan ricotta cheese

1 1/2 cups shredded vegan mozzarella cheese

Finely chopped fresh parsley and basil, for topping

Instructions

Preheat the oven to 375° F. Combine 6 tablespoons olive oil and the garlic in a large pot or Dutch oven over medium-high heat. Cook, stirring, until golden brown, 2 to 3 minutes. Stir in the oregano and red pepper flakes, then add the tomatoes. Bring to a boil, then reduce the heat to maintain a steady simmer. Add 1 teaspoon salt and a few grinds of pepper and cook, stirring occasionally, until slightly thickened, about 10 minutes. (The sauce will thicken further as the pasta bakes.) Taste and adjust the seasoning with salt and pepper.

Meanwhile, bring a large pot of salted water to a boil. Add the pasta and cook as the label directs for al dente. Reserve 1 cup cooking water, then drain.

While the pasta cooks, heat the remaining 3 tablespoons olive oil in a large skillet over medium-high heat. Add the mushrooms and season with salt and pepper. Cook, undisturbed, until the mushrooms start to brown, about 4 minutes. Stir and continue cooking until lightly browned all over and the skillet is mostly dry, 3 to 4 more minutes. Add the mushrooms to the tomato sauce.

Add the cooked pasta to the tomato sauce and toss, adding the reserved cooking water, 1/4 cup at a time, as needed to loosen (it should be saucy). Spread about half of the pasta in a 9-by-13-inch baking dish. Dot with half of the ricotta, then top with the remaining pasta and sauce. Dot with the remaining ricotta, then scatter the mozzarella all over. Bake until the sauce is bubbling and the cheese warms and softens, 15 to 20 minutes (vegan mozzarella will not melt and spread like dairy cheese). Let stand at least 10 minutes. Sprinkle with parsley and basil and drizzle with olive oil.

Malai Kofta

Ingredients

Kofta:

Yukon gold potatoes (about 10 ounces), boiled, drained and mashed

1/2 cup fresh cilantro leaves and tender stems, chopped

1 small Thai green chile or 1/2 serrano pepper, seeded and chopped

Kosher salt and freshly ground black pepper

3 ounces paneer, cubed

3 tablespoons mixed nuts, such as pistachios, cashews, pine nuts and/or almonds

2 tablespoons dried fruit, such as raisins, currants, barberries and/or cranberries

1/2 cup besan (fine chickpea flour)

Vegetable oil, for frying

Sauce:

3/4 teaspoon garam masala

1/2 teaspoon Kashmiri chili powder

1/2 teaspoon ground coriander

1/4 teaspoon ground turmeric

2 tablespoons extra-virgin olive oil or vegetable oil

1 tablespoon unsalted butter

1/2 teaspoon cumin seeds

1 large onion, coarsely chopped

1 1/2 teaspoons grated garlic

1 1/2 teaspoons grated ginger

Kosher salt

1/4 cup raw cashews, soaked in hot water for at least
30 minutes

3/4 cup canned whole peeled tomatoes, such as San
Marzanos, crushed by hand

1/4 cup heavy cream

1/4 teaspoon kasoori methi (dried fenugreek
leaves), gently crushed by hand, optional

Serving:

1/4 teaspoon garam masala

Fresh cilantro leaves, for serving

Instructions

Special equipment: a deep-fry thermometer; a kitchen scale, optional

For the kofta:

Combine the mashed potatoes, cilantro, chiles, 1 teaspoon salt and 1/4 teaspoon pepper in a large bowl. Knead the mixture until thoroughly combined. Taste and adjust the seasoning, then set aside.

Put the paneer in a food processor and pulse until crumbly. Add the nuts and dried fruit and pulse until the fruit is coarsely chopped and the nuts are broken into small pieces. (If the paneer is not salted, add a pinch of salt.) Transfer the paneer mixture to a small bowl.

Form the mashed potato mixture into 8 equal balls. (A kitchen scale isn't necessary, but is helpful.) Form the paneer mixture into 8 equal balls. They don't have to be perfectly shaped, but it is much easier to stuff the potato balls when the paneer mixture has been squished into little balls.

Hold a potato ball in the palm of your hand. Make an indentation with your thumb. Place a paneer ball into the concave hollow and push it in gently. Pinch the potato mixture around it and roll the potato ball in your palm to make a nice round shape. Repeat with the remaining potato and paneer balls. If the potato mixture is sticking to your hands and preventing you from rolling a smooth ball, dampen the palms of your hands with a little room-temperature water and continue rolling.

Place the besan in a shallow bowl. Gently roll the stuffed balls in the besan. Transfer the coated balls to a plate, cover with plastic wrap and refrigerate while you make the sauce. (It is easier to fry the balls when they have rested and are cold.)

For the sauce:

Meanwhile, stir together the garam masala, Kashmiri chili powder, coriander, turmeric and 2 tablespoons water in a small bowl until combined. Set the spice mixture aside.

Heat the olive oil and butter in a medium saucepan over medium heat. Add the cumin seeds and let sizzle until they darken slightly, about 30 seconds. Add the onions and cook, stirring occasionally, until softened and just starting to get a hint of color, 8 to 10 minutes. (Do not brown them, as that will affect the color of the sauce.)

Add the garlic, ginger and 1/2 teaspoon salt, mix well and cook, stirring often, until the raw smell goes away, about 2 minutes. Add the spice mixture and cook, stirring often, until the oil comes out, about 5 minutes.

Drain the cashews and add to the saucepan, then add the tomatoes and 1/2 teaspoon salt. Increase the heat to medium high and cook until the tomato mixture is thickened and pasty, about 7 minutes. Set aside and let cool.

Meanwhile, fry the kofta. Fill a large Dutch oven halfway with vegetable oil, attach a deep-fry thermometer and heat over medium-high heat to 350 degrees F. Set a cooling rack over a baking sheet and place a paper towel over the rack. Carefully add half the balls, one at a time, and fry, turning occasionally, until golden brown, about 3 minutes.

Using a slotted spoon, remove the balls to the prepared rack. Repeat with the remaining balls.

Transfer the cooled sauce to a blender, add 1 cup water and process until smooth. Transfer the sauce back to the saucepan. Add the cream and kasoori methi if using and heat over medium heat until simmering. It should have the consistency of a smooth carrot soup; Add more water, if needed, and adjust the salt to taste.

Gently add the fried kofta and heat, occasionally shaking the pan gently to coat the balls, until hot, about 3 minutes.

For serving:

Garnish with the garam masala and cilantro leaves.

Falafel

Ingredients

Vegetable oil, for frying

8 ounces dried chickpeas, soaked overnight, drained and rinsed

3/4 cup fresh parsley leaves

1 1/2 teaspoons baking powder dissolved in 3 tablespoons water

1 teaspoon ground cumin

1/2 teaspoon ground coriander

1/8 teaspoon cayenne pepper

1 clove garlic, chopped

1 small onion, chopped

Kosher salt

Serving suggestions: pita bread, lettuce, tomato, tahini, hot sauce and lemon wedges

Instructions

Special equipment: a deep-frying thermometer

Heat 3 inches oil in large heavy pot to 365 degrees F.

Add the drained chickpeas to a food processor. Pulse until the chickpeas begin to break down, about 30 seconds. Add the parsley, baking powder and water, cumin, coriander, cayenne, garlic, onion and 2 teaspoons salt. Process continuously, stopping to scrape down the bowl once halfway through, until a homogenous paste forms, about 2 minutes.

Using a 1-ounce cookie scoop or 2 tablespoons, scoop the falafel mixture into balls and carefully drop one at a time into the hot oil in batches of nine. Fry until very deep golden brown all over, 1 1/2 to 2 minutes. Use a spider or slotted spoon to transfer the falafel to a paper towel-lined plate or wire rack-lined baking sheet to drain. Repeat the process with the remaining mixture.

Serve the warm falafel with pita bread, lettuce, tomato, tahini, hot sauce and lemon wedges.

Lentil-Mushroom Meatballs

Ingredients

Sauce:

2 tablespoons extra-virgin olive oil

4 cloves garlic, thinly sliced

One 28-ounce can whole peeled tomatoes, crushed by hand

Small handful torn fresh basil leaves

Kosher salt

Meatballs:

3 tablespoons extra-virgin olive oil, plus more for brushing the baking sheet

1/3 cup wheat berries

1 cup dry brown lentils, rinsed and sorted

1 small yellow onion, finely chopped

4 ounces shiitake mushrooms, stemmed and roughly chopped

5 cloves garlic, finely chopped

Kosher salt and freshly ground black pepper

3 tablespoons tomato paste

3 tablespoons low-sodium soy sauce

2 tablespoons red wine vinegar

4 teaspoons nutritional yeast

1/2 cup fresh parsley leaves, plus more for garnish

2 slices white bread or 1 hamburger bun, torn into small pieces

Instructions

For the sauce:

Put the oil and garlic in a medium saucepan over medium heat. Swirl until the garlic is just lightly browned and fragrant, about 4 minutes. Add the tomatoes and 1/2 cup water. Bring to a high simmer, then reduce the heat to medium-low. Add the torn basil leaves and 2 teaspoons salt and simmer, uncovered, until thickened, 20 to 25 minutes.

For the meatballs:

Meanwhile, preheat the oven to 400 degrees F. Line a baking sheet with parchment paper and brush with oil.

Bring a medium saucepan of water to a boil, then add the wheat berries and boil until plump and tender, about 30 minutes. Drain and set aside.

Put the lentils in a medium saucepan with 2 1/2 cups water. Bring to a boil, then reduce heat to low and simmer, uncovered, until almost all of the water has evaporated and the lentils are soft, about 15 minutes. Remove from the heat, drain and let cool slightly.

Meanwhile, heat the oil in a large nonstick skillet over medium heat. Add the onion, mushrooms, garlic, 1 teaspoon salt and a few grinds of pepper and cook, stirring until soft and lightly browned, about 6 minutes. Add the tomato paste, soy sauce, vinegar and nutritional yeast and cook, stirring, until the liquid has evaporated and is slightly dry, about 2 more minutes. Let cool slightly. Clean out the skillet.

Transfer the onion-mushroom mixture to a food processor. Add the cooked lentils, wheat berries and parsley leaves. Pulse until the mixture is combined and crumbly but not mushy.

Put the torn bread into a large bowl and cover with 1/4 cup of water. Let sit at least 5 minutes to soften. Using a fork, mash the soaked bread into a paste. Add the lentil mixture to the bowl with the mashed bread and mix by hand until fully incorporated. The mixture should hold its shape when squeezed gently.

Shape the mixture by hand into 18 golf-ball sized meatballs. Place about 1 inch apart on the prepared baking sheet. Bake until the meatballs are golden brown on the outside and don't crumble when gently pressed, 25 to 30 minutes.

To serve, pour the sauce into a shallow serving bowl. Put the hot meatballs on top of the sauce and garnish with parsley.

RECIPES FOR LUNCH ON THE HASHIMOTO'S VEGETARIAN DIET

Crustless Caprese Quiche

Ingredients

Nonstick cooking spray

1/3 cup plus 2 tablespoons whole wheat or other whole grain breadcrumbs

2 teaspoons extra-virgin olive oil

1 medium onion, diced

Kosher salt

4 plum tomatoes (2 chopped and 2 thinly sliced crosswise)

2 large eggs plus 2 large egg whites

1/2 cup part-skim ricotta cheese

1/2 cup 2-percent milk

1/4 cup packed fresh basil leaves, thinly sliced, plus 1 sprig for garnish

4 ounces shredded part-skim mozzarella

Instructions

Preheat the oven to 350 degrees F. Coat a 9-inch deep-sided pie pan with nonstick cooking spray. Evenly sprinkle 2 tablespoons of the breadcrumbs into the pan.

Heat the oil in a large nonstick skillet over medium-low heat. Add the onion and 1/8 teaspoon salt and cover the skillet. Cook, stirring occasionally, until the onions soften without color, about 15 minutes. Stir in the chopped tomatoes and cook for 1 minute. Transfer to a medium bowl and set aside.

Meanwhile, add the eggs, egg whites, ricotta, milk, the remaining 1/3 cup breadcrumbs and 3/4 teaspoon salt to a blender until well combined and smooth. Stir in the sliced basil and the onion-tomato mixture.

Pour the egg mixture into the prepared pie pan. Sprinkle with the mozzarella. Arrange the sliced tomatoes in an overlapping style around the top.

Bake until the eggs are set and the cheese is lightly browned, about 35 minutes. Let stand for 10 minutes to complete the cooking process. Garnish with the fresh basil sprig. Slice into 4 wedges with a sharp knife and serve.

Air Fryer Chili-Garlic Tofu with Green Beans

Ingredients

Two 14-ounce packages extra-firm tofu

2 tablespoons olive oil

Kosher salt and freshly ground black pepper

1 pound green beans, trimmed

1/3 cup low-sodium soy sauce

2 tablespoons rice wine vinegar

2 tablespoons mirin

1 heaping tablespoon brown sugar

1 to 2 teaspoons chili-garlic paste or sambal (add amount to spice level preference)

1 teaspoon cornstarch

3 cloves garlic, smashed whole

2 scallions, thinly sliced

Instructions

Special equipment: a 6-quart air fryer

Drain the tofu, wrap each block in several layers of paper towel and set on a large plate. Place a heavy pan on top (cast-iron works great for this) to press excess liquid from the tofu; allow to rest for 15 minutes.

Slice each tofu block into six 1/2-inch-thick slices. Drain the large plate of any excess liquid, wipe dry and place the tofu slices back on the plate. Put 1 tablespoon of the oil in a small bowl and use a pastry brush to coat both sides of the slices with the oil. Season both sides of the slices with 1 teaspoon salt and several grinds of pepper.

Preheat the air fryer to 400 degrees F.

Lay the tofu slices flat in the basket of the air fryer and cook, flipping halfway through, until lightly golden and crisp, about 20 minutes. Transfer to a plate.

Preheat the air fryer to 400 degrees F again.

Toss the green beans in a large bowl with the remaining 1 tablespoon oil, 1/2 teaspoon salt and several grinds of pepper. Cook the beans, tossing halfway through, until tender and blistered, about 10 minutes.

While the beans cook, combine the soy sauce, rice wine vinegar, mirin, brown sugar, chili-garlic paste, cornstarch, garlic and 3 tablespoons water in a small saucepan and stir until the cornstarch is dissolved. Cook over medium-low heat, stirring occasionally, until the sauce is slightly reduced, thickened and shiny, 5 to 7 minutes.

Transfer the beans to a large serving plate and shingle the tofu slices on top. Drizzle the sauce over the tofu and beans and garnish with the scallions.

Whole Cauliflower Wellington

Ingredients

1/4 cup fresh flat-leaf parsley leaves, chopped

1 tablespoon fresh thyme leaves, chopped

Kosher salt and freshly ground black pepper

8 tablespoons (1 stick) unsalted butter, at room temperature

1 large cauliflower (about 3 pounds)

1 pound cremini mushrooms, stems trimmed

Two sheets frozen puff pastry (from a 17.3-ounce package), thawed

2 tablespoons Dijon mustard

1 large egg, beaten

Instructions

Preheat the oven to 400 degrees F. Line a baking with parchment.

Combine the parsley, thyme, 1/2 teaspoon salt and a few grinds of pepper in to a food processor and process until finely chopped. Add the butter and process until well combined and the butter is very green. Clean out the food processor.

Carefully remove the leaves and any small inner leave from the bottom of the cauliflower and trim the stem so it is 1/2-inch-long. Brush the cauliflower with 2 tablespoons of the herb butter and sprinkle with 1/2 teaspoon salt and a few grinds of pepper. Transfer to the prepared baking sheet and bake until a paring knife can easily be inserted and removed from stalk and the cauliflower has turned a light golden brown, 25 to 30 minutes.

Meanwhile, pulse the mushrooms in a food processor until a paste. Melt 2 tablespoons of the herb butter in a large nonstick skillet over medium-high heat. Add the mushroom paste, 1 teaspoon salt and a few grinds of pepper and cook, stirring occasionally, until all the moisture has evaporated, about 10 minutes. Let cool slightly, about 10 minutes.

Place 1 puff pastry sheet on top of the other. Roll out to a 14-by-14-inch square with a 3-inch-wide border all the way around that is considerably thinner than the middle. Round the corners so you have a 13-inch circle. Brush the puff pastry with the Dijon, then spread the mushroom mixture over top. Turn the cauliflower upside down on top of and in the middle of the puff pastry circle. Melt the remaining herb butter in the microwave in 30 second intervals. Pour the butter in between the stalks of the florets. Fold the puff pastry around the cauliflower so that the whole thing is enclosed. Turn the cauliflower right side up, place it back onto the prepared baking sheet and brush with the egg. Sprinkle with 1/2 teaspoon salt and bake until the puff pastry is a deep golden brown and a paring knife can be easily inserted, twisted and removed from the stem of the cauliflower, 55 to 60 minutes. Let cool for 10 minutes before serving. Slice through the middle then into wedges.

Menemen

Ingredients

2 tablespoons olive oil

1 Italian sweet pepper, such as cubanelle, diced

4 large tomatoes (about 1 1/2 pounds), diced

3 large eggs

Kosher salt and freshly ground black pepper

1/4 cup fresh parsley, chopped, optional

Warm bread, for serving

Instructions

Heat the olive oil in a large pan over medium heat. Saute the sweet pepper, stirring frequently, until it softens, about 5 minutes. Add the tomatoes and cook, stirring occasionally, until they start breaking down and releasing their juices, 5 to 8 minutes.

Break the eggs into a small bowl and beat lightly using a fork. Add the eggs to the tomatoes and stir to combine. Add 1/2 teaspoon salt and about 1/3 teaspoon black pepper. Cook, gently stirring, until the eggs are just set, about 3 minutes, making sure not to overcook the eggs. Garnish with parsley if using and serve with warm bread.

Buckwheat Noodle Salad

Ingredients

1/4 cup plus 2 tablespoons rice vinegar

1 teaspoon sugar

2 tablespoons peeled and finely grated fresh ginger

1 tablespoon honey

2 tablespoons tamari

2 teaspoons toasted sesame oil

2 teaspoons chili sauce (recommended: Sriracha)

1/4 cup canola oil

12 ounces buckwheat noodles, cooked according to package directions, rinsed under cold water and drained

1 carrot, peeled and grated on box grater

1 red bell pepper, seeded and julienned

1/4 English cucumber, peeled and grated on a box grater

3 green onions, thinly sliced

1/4 cup chopped fresh cilantro leaves

Instructions

Whisk together the vinegar, sugar, ginger, honey, tamari, sesame oil, and chili sauce in a large bowl until combined. Slowly whisk in the canola oil until the dressing is emulsified.

Add the noodles, carrot, pepper, cucumber, green onions and cilantro. Gently mix to combine and serve.

Papeta par Eda

Ingredients

4 tablespoons extra-virgin olive oil or vegetable oil

3 red onions (about 1 pound), thinly sliced

1 tablespoon peeled and grated fresh ginger

1 to 5 Thai green chiles or 1 to 2 serrano peppers (depending on your spice level), finely chopped

3 cloves garlic, grated

1 tablespoon unsalted butter

3 Yukon gold potatoes (about 1 pound), peeled, cut into approximately 1/8-inch slices and soaked in a large bowl of water

Kosher salt and freshly ground pepper

1/2 cup chopped fresh cilantro leaves and tender stems

6 large eggs

Instructions

Special equipment: a heavy skillet with a lid

Heat the oil in a large heavy skillet over medium-high heat. Add the onions and cook, stirring occasionally, until soft, 4 to 5 minutes. Add the ginger, chiles and garlic and cook, stirring occasionally, until the raw smell goes away, about 3 minutes.

Add the butter, potatoes and 2 teaspoons salt and gently stir to combine. Lower the heat to medium and cook, occasionally gently turning over the potato and onion mixture from the bottom, until the potatoes are just cooked, but still firm, about 10 minutes. Some of the potatoes should have nice crispy edges and some of the onions should be caramelized.

Add most of the cilantro (reserving some for garnish) and gently stir in. Adjust the salt to taste. Gently flatten out the mixture and make 6 evenly spaced nests in it using the back of a spoon. Crack an egg into each nest.

Pour 2 tablespoons of water around the edge of the skillet. Cover the skillet, lower the heat to medium-low and cook until the egg whites are set and the yolks are still slightly wobbly, 8 to 10 minutes. (Open the lid and peek every few minutes to make sure the eggs are not getting overcooked.)

Sprinkle with some salt and pepper and garnish with the remaining cilantro.

Vegan Black Bean Enchiladas

Ingredients

1 tablespoon olive oil

1 teaspoon chili powder

1 teaspoon ground cumin

2 cloves garlic, minced

1 small onion, chopped

Kosher salt and freshly ground black pepper

1 tablespoon tomato paste

One 15-ounce can diced tomatoes

1 canned chipotle in adobo, chopped, plus 1 teaspoon adobo sauce

One 15-ounce can black beans, drained and rinsed

1 cup frozen corn

10 corn tortillas

One 19-ounce can vegan red enchilada sauce

16 slices vegan Cheddar (about 12 ounces)

Fresh cilantro leaves, chopped avocado, sliced radishes and hot sauce, for topping

Instructions

Preheat the oven to 400 degrees F.

Heat the olive oil in a large skillet over medium-high heat. Add the chili powder, cumin, garlic, onion, 1 teaspoon salt and a few grinds of pepper and cook, stirring occasionally, until the onion is softened, 5 to 6 minutes. Add the tomato paste and cook, stirring to combine, until the tomato paste is a deep brick red, 3 to 4 minutes. Add the diced tomatoes and chipotle with the adobo sauce and cook, stirring occasionally and mashing the tomatoes with a wooden spoon, until the sauce is thickened and reduced by a quarter, about 6 minutes. Add the beans, corn, 1/2 teaspoon salt and a few grinds of pepper and cook just until the beans and corn are warmed through, 3 to 4 minutes.

Microwave the tortillas so they are just warmed and more pliable, about 30 seconds. Spread 1/2 cup of the enchilada sauce on the bottom of a 13-by-9-inch baking dish. Pour the remaining enchilada sauce into a large shallow bowl or pie dish.

Dip each tortilla into the bowl of enchilada sauce to lightly coat. Place 1 slice of Cheddar inside each tortilla and fill with 2 heaping tablespoons of the black bean mixture. Fold the tortillas over the filling and transfer to the baking dish. Pour the remaining enchilada sauce over top of the tortillas and lay the remaining 6 cheese slices on top down the middle.

Bake until the cheese has melted and is turning brown in spots and the edges of the tortillas start to crisp, 15 to 20 minutes. Garnish with cilantro, avocado, radishes and hot sauce.

Chipotle-Inspired Vegetarian Burrito Bowl

Ingredients

1 small onion, one half cut into thick wedges through the stem and the other half finely diced

1 medium poblano chile

3 tablespoons olive oil

1 chipotle pepper and 2 tablespoons adobo sauce (from one 7-ounce can chipotle peppers in adobo sauce)

2 cloves garlic

2 teaspoons low-sodium soy sauce

2 teaspoons tomato paste

1 teaspoon chili powder

1 teaspoon red wine vinegar

1/2 teaspoon ground cumin

Kosher salt and freshly ground black pepper

One 14-ounce package extra-firm tofu, drained well

Brown rice, for serving

Black beans, for serving

Shredded romaine lettuce, for serving

Prepared pico de gallo, for serving

Instructions

Preheat the oven to broil.

Place the onion wedges and poblano on a rimmed
baking sheet and rub with 1 tablespoon of the olive

oil. Broil, turning several times with tongs, until the poblano has collapsed in on itself and the vegetables are charred, 6 to 8 minutes. Remove from the oven. When the poblano is cool enough to handle, remove and discard the skin, stem and seeds.

Transfer the poblano to a blender. Add the charred onion wedges, chipotle pepper and adobo sauce, garlic, soy sauce, tomato paste, chili powder, vinegar, cumin, 1/2 cup water, 3/4 teaspoon salt and a few grinds of pepper. Blend until smooth, then set the poblano mixture aside.

Cut the tofu crosswise into 1/4-inch-thick planks, then press the pieces between a couple paper towels to remove as much moisture as possible. Heat 1 tablespoon of the olive oil in a large nonstick skillet over medium-high heat. Add the tofu and cook until well browned, about 5 minutes per side. Transfer to a plate to cool.

Heat the remaining 1 tablespoon olive oil in the same skillet, then add the diced onions and cook, stirring occasionally, until tender, about 6 minutes. Using your hands, tear and crumble the tofu into very small pieces and add to the skillet. Cook, stirring to combine, until warmed through, about 2 minutes.

Add the poblano mixture and 1/2 cup water to the skillet and cook until it's bubbling all over and the tofu has absorbed some of the sauce, about 5 minutes. Add 1 to 2 more tablespoons water if the mixture gets too dry (it should be saucy). Taste and add more salt and pepper, if needed.

Serve over rice and beans and top with lettuce and pico de gallo.

Buddha's Delight

Ingredients

3 ounces dried bean curd sticks, broken into 2-inch pieces

2/3 cup dried wood ear mushrooms (2 ounces)

12 medium dried shiitake mushrooms (2 ounces)

Two 3-ounces packages cellophane noodles (also called bean thread vermicelli)

2 tablespoons light soy sauce

1 tablespoon plus 1 teaspoon oyster sauce (or use vegetarian oyster sauce if you prefer)

2 teaspoons sugar

1 teaspoon dark soy sauce

1/4 teaspoon ground white pepper

2 tablespoons Shaoxing wine

Kosher salt

1 1/2 ounces red fermented bean curd (hong fu yu; about 3 pieces)

2 tablespoons vegetable, canola or peanut oil

1 1/2 teaspoons finely minced ginger

3 cloves garlic, finely minced

1/2 medium head napa cabbage (about 1 1/2 pounds), core discarded, cut into 1-inch pieces, leafy parts and thick stems separated

4 ounces snow peas or sugar snap peas, stemmed and strings removed

1 teaspoon toasted sesame oil

Instructions

Soak the bean curd sticks and wood ear mushrooms in a large bowl of hot water at room temperature until the bean curd sticks are just hydrated, about 1 hour. Drain and rinse under cold water, then drain again. Cut off the tough stems from the wood ear mushrooms and discard; cut the mushrooms into bite-size pieces. Set aside with the bean curd sticks.

Soak the shiitake mushrooms in a medium bowl of hot water at room temperature until rehydrated, about 1 hour. Remove the shiitakes from the soaking liquid, then pour the liquid through a fine-mesh strainer into a measuring cup and add enough cold water if needed until it measures 2/3 cup. Cut off and discard the stems of the shiitake mushrooms, then slice the mushrooms into 1/2-inch pieces. Set aside.

Soak the cellophane noodles in a separate medium bowl with warm water until softened, about 30 minutes. Drain the noodles and set aside.

Mix the light soy sauce, oyster sauce, sugar, dark soy sauce, white pepper, 1 tablespoon of the Shaoxing wine and 1/2 teaspoon salt in a small bowl until the sugar is dissolved. Smash the red fermented bean curd into a paste in a separate small bowl. Set aside.

Bring a medium pot of water to a boil over high heat. Blanch the wood ear mushrooms and bean curd sticks until the bean curd sticks are softened, about 3 minutes. Drain and set aside.

Heat a wok over medium heat until it starts to smoke, about 2 minutes. Add the vegetable oil and heat until shimmering. Stir-fry the ginger and garlic until fragrant, about 10 seconds. Add the red fermented bean curd (set aside the bowl for later use) and stir-fry until broken down further and fragrant, about 1 minute. Add the shiitake mushrooms and napa cabbage stems and cook until the cabbage starts to soften and the red of the bean curd darkens, about 2 minutes.

Deglaze with the remaining tablespoon Shaoxing, then add most of the reserved 2/3 cup mushroom-soaking liquid (hold back a couple tablespoons) and bring to a boil, covered, over high heat. Once boiling, add the wood ear mushrooms and bean curd sticks, cover and cook over high heat until the cabbage stems are just tender, about 4 minutes.

Add the reserved sauce, then stir some of the remaining mushroom-soaking liquid into the sauce bowl and the rest into the reserved red fermented bean curd bowl to dissolve any remaining sauce or bean curd, then add to the wok and stir until combined. Taste the liquid for seasoning and add more salt if needed. Shift the vegetables up the wok and add the cellophane noodles and cabbage leaves.

Stir to submerge the noodles and cook, covered, until the noodles are softened, about 2 minutes.

Uncover and toss the noodles to evenly coat in the sauce. Add the snow peas and toss so they are distributed under the hot vegetables to cook slightly. Drizzle over the toasted sesame oil and toss until combined.

Vegetarian Chili

Ingredients

1 (28-ounce) can diced tomatoes

4 cups reduced-sodium vegetable broth

1 (15-ounce) can black beans, rinsed and drained

1 (15-ounce) can white (cannellini) beans, rinsed and drained

1 (15-ounce) can red kidney beans, rinsed and drained

1 cup frozen baby lima beans or regular lima beans

1 cup chopped onion

1 green bell pepper, seeded and chopped

2 cloves garlic, minced

1 tablespoon minced pickled jalapeno (from can or jar)

2 tablespoons chili powder

2 tablespoons dried Mexican oregano or regular oregano

2 teaspoons ground cumin

1 teaspoon ground coriander

1 to 2 teaspoons hot sauce

1/3 cup couscous

1/2 cup shredded Monterey jack cheese

1/3 cup chopped fresh cilantro leaves

Salt and freshly ground black pepper

Instructions

In a slow cooker, combine all ingredients but the couscous, shredded cheese, cilantro and salt and pepper. Cover and cook on LOW for 6 to 8 hours or on HIGH for 3 to 4 hours.

Five to 10 minutes before serving (depending on temperature of slow cooker) add couscous, cover and cook, until couscous is tender. Season, to taste, with salt and black pepper.

Just before serving, top each serving with shredded cheese and cilantro.

Cauliflower Parmesan

Ingredients

1 medium head cauliflower

1 cup all-purpose flour

Kosher salt

3 large eggs, beaten

2 cups panko breadcrumbs

About 1 cup olive oil

2 1/2 cups marinara sauce, from a 24-ounce jar

1/2 pound fresh mozzarella, thinly sliced

1/3 cup grated Parmesan

1/4 cup torn fresh basil leaves

Instructions

Preheat the oven to 400 degrees F and line a plate with paper towels.

Pull off the leaves from the base of the cauliflower and cut off the stem, but do not cut out the core. Slice the cauliflower into 1-inch thick slices, aiming for about 3 nice "steaks" from the center. The rest will break into smaller florets, and that is okay.

Mix the flour with 1 teaspoon salt in a shallow bowl or pie plate. Put the eggs in another shallow bowl and panko in a third shallow bowl.

Add 1/4 inch olive oil to a large skillet and heat over medium-high heat until shimmering.

Working with the larger pieces first, add the cauliflower to the flour and turn to coat. Shake off the excess, then dip in the egg to coat. Let the excess egg drip off, then coat thoroughly in the panko. Fry the cauliflower in batches to avoid overcrowding, turning once, until golden brown on both sides, 6 to 8 minutes total. Transfer to the lined plate to drain and sprinkle with salt. Repeat with the remaining smaller pieces of cauliflower (leave out any tiny crumbly pieces).

Spread 1 cup marinara sauce on the bottom of a 9-by-13-inch baking dish. Arrange the fried cauliflower on top, then spoon 1 cup of the sauce on top of the cauliflower. Arrange the mozzarella over the sauce, then spoon the remaining 1/2 cup marinara over the top. Sprinkle with the Parmesan and bake until bubbling and lightly browned in spots, about 35 minutes. Sprinkle with the basil and serve.

Lentil Frittata

Ingredients

1 cup green lentils

Kosher salt and freshly ground black pepper

3 tablespoons olive oil

1 onion, diced

3 cloves garlic

1 russet potato, diced very small

2 cups baby spinach, chopped

10 large eggs

1/2 cup milk

1 teaspoon crushed red pepper flakes (less if you don't like it to be a bit spicy)

1 cup crumbled feta

Chopped kalamata and green olives, chopped fresh parsley, sliced tomato and olive oil, for toppings

Instructions

Cook the lentils with 1 teaspoon salt and 1/2 teaspoon black pepper with 2 cups of water in a medium saucepan over medium-high heat until fully cooked but not mushy, 25 to 30 minutes. Drain lentils of excess water in a fine sieve and let them come to room temperature.

Meanwhile, preheat the oven to 400 degrees F. Heat the olive oil in a large (12-inch) seasoned cast-iron skillet over medium heat. Sauté the onion, stirring frequently, until soft and translucent, about 10 minutes. Add in the garlic and finely diced potato and sauté, stirring often, until the potatoes start to soften a bit, about 15 minutes. Add the spinach and cook, tossing, until wilted but still vibrant green, about 5 minutes. Add the cooked lentils and 1 teaspoon salt and stir.

Whisk the eggs in a large bowl, then mix in the milk, red pepper flakes and half of the feta. Pour over the vegetables in the skillet and gently stir to combine. Then top with the rest of the feta and bake until the eggs are set, 20 to 25 minutes. If desired, turn on the broiler for 3 to 5 minutes to brown the top.

Top with some chopped olives and parsley, tomato slices and a good drizzle of olive oil.

Note: It's best to purchase a block of feta and crumble it yourself since it'll keep its moisture and taste much better. As for the milk, you can use whole milk, 2% or even dairy-free milk if desired.

Vegan Chickpea Crab Cakes

Ingredients

Chickpea Crab Cakes:

Two 15-ounce cans chickpeas, drained and 1/4 cup liquid reserved

Pinch cream of tartar

2 tablespoons fresh parsley, chopped

1 tablespoon lemon juice, plus lemon wedges for serving

2 teaspoons Old Bay Seasoning

1 teaspoon honey mustard

2 slices of white bread or 1 hamburger bun, torn into small pieces

Kosher salt

2/3 cup all-purpose flour

Vegetable oil, for frying

Tartar Sauce:

1/4 cup vegan mayonnaise

1/2 teaspoon honey mustard

Pinch Old Bay Seasoning

1/2 whole dill pickle, finely chopped

1 tablespoon dill pickle brine

Instructions

For the chickpea crab cakes: Place the reserved chickpea liquid into a large bowl, then add the cream of tartar and whip vigorously until foamy and thick.

Whisk in the parsley, lemon juice, Old Bay and honey mustard, then add the bread pieces and toss to coat. Let sit until the bread is soft, about 5 minutes.

Meanwhile, finely chop the chickpeas (alternatively, you can pinch or smush them). When the bread mixture is ready, add the chickpeas and toss and squeeze the mixture until it holds together. Form into eight 3/4-inch thick patties with nice rounded edges. Cover and chill them for at least 1 hour.

For the tartar sauce: Whisk together the mayonnaise, honey mustard, Old Bay, pickle and pickle brine in a small bowl. Refrigerate until ready to serve.

Preheat the oven to 350 degrees F. Whisk a large pinch of salt into the flour and put on a plate. Pour enough oil to cover the bottom of a large nonstick skillet and heat over medium-high heat. Dredge half of the cakes in the flour. Once the oil is hot and

149

shimmering, add the cakes and cook until crunchy and deep golden brown, about 3 minutes per side. Adjust the heat as necessary to keep them from browning too quickly. Transfer to a baking sheet and repeat with the remaining cakes. Sprinkle each with salt, then bake until heated completely through, about 5 minutes.

Serve the chickpea crab cakes with the tartar sauce and lemon wedges.

Vegetarian Chicken-Fried Portobello Mushroom Steaks

Ingredients

1 cup milk

2 large eggs

Vegetable oil, for frying

Mashed potatoes, for serving

Vegetarian Gravy, recipe follows, heated

4 extra-large Portobello mushrooms, stemmed (do not remove gills)

Kosher salt

1 1/2 cups all-purpose flour

2 teaspoons baking powder

Freshly ground black pepper

Sliced fresh chives or scallions, for garnish, optional

Vegetarian Gravy:

1 medium onion, quartered

2 stalks celery, roughly chopped

1 medium carrot, roughly chopped

3 cloves garlic, crushed

1 teaspoon vegetable oil

Kosher salt

1 ounce dried shiitake mushrooms (about 1 heaping cup)

6 sprigs thyme

2 sun-dried tomatoes

2 tablespoons low-sodium soy sauce

1 dried bay leaf

4 tablespoons unsalted butter

6 fresh sage leaves

1/3 cup all-purpose flour

1/4 cup chopped fresh parsley

Freshly ground black pepper

Instructions

Special equipment: A deep-fry thermometer

Position an oven rack at the top of the oven, and preheat the broiler. Arrange the mushrooms on a baking sheet, and broil until the sides facing up begin to soften, about 5 minutes. Flip, and continue to broil until the sides facing up are soft, about 5 minutes more. Let cool.

Put the mushrooms, gill-side up, between 2 pieces of plastic wrap, and pound to about 1/4 inch thick with a meat mallet. Season all over with 1/2 teaspoon salt.

Whisk together the flour, baking powder and 1 teaspoon each salt and pepper in a shallow dish. Whisk together the milk and eggs in a separate shallow dish.

Lower the oven heat to 250 degrees F. Put a rack over a rimmed baking sheet. Heat about an inch of oil to 350 degrees F in a large cast-iron skillet or Dutch oven over medium-high heat.

While the oil heats, dredge each mushroom in the flour mixture to completely coat; shake off any excess. Then dip into the egg mixture until fully coated; let the excess drip off. Return the mushroom to the flour mixture, and dredge a second time, until completely coated, pressing firmly into the flour mixture. Arrange on one side of the rack on the baking sheet.

Add 2 of the breaded mushrooms to the hot oil, and cook, turning once, until crisp and golden, about 5 minutes total. Transfer the mushrooms to the unused side of the rack. When the oil comes back to temperature, repeat with the remaining 2 mushrooms and keep the first 2 warm in the oven.

Serve the mushroom steaks with mashed potatoes and generous spoonful's of hot gravy. Garnish with chives or scallions if using.

Vegetarian Gravy:

Yield: 2 1/2 cups

Position an oven rack in the top position in the oven and preheat to 450 degrees F. Toss the onions, celery, carrots and garlic with the oil and 1 teaspoon salt on a rimmed baking sheet. Roast until the vegetables are charred in some places, 25 to 30 minutes.

Bring the roasted vegetables, 1 cup water, mushrooms, thyme, sun-dried tomatoes, soy sauce, bay leaf and 1 teaspoon salt to a simmer in a medium saucepan over medium-high heat. Cook, stirring occasionally, until most of the liquid is gone, 8 to 10 minutes. Add 6 cups water and 1/2 teaspoon salt, and bring back to a simmer. Reduce the heat to medium-low, and gently simmer until reduced by about one third, about 45 minutes. Strain the stock into a large liquid measuring cup, then squeeze all the liquid out of the solids with the back of a ladle (there should be about 4 cups of stock); discard the solids. (If not making gravy right away, let the stock cool to room temperature, then refrigerate for up to 3 days or freeze for up to 1 month; warm slightly before making gravy.)

Melt the butter in a medium saucepan over medium heat. Add the sage leaves to the butter, and stir for 30 seconds; remove the fried sage leaves, and set aside. Add the flour to the saucepan, and stir until smooth and lightly golden, about 2 minutes. Slowly pour in the warm stock while whisking constantly until smooth and thick, 8 to 10 minutes.

Chop the fried sage, stir it and the parsley into the gravy and season to taste with pepper.

Shortcut Chana Masala

Ingredients

Two 15-ounce cans chickpeas, rinsed well and drained

2 bay leaves

1 black tea bag (or 2 teaspoons black tea in a muslin bag)

1 black cardamom pod, optional

Kosher salt

4 tablespoons ghee or oil (I like to use a combination of both)

2 medium onions, chopped (about 1 3/4 cups)

2 inches ginger, peeled and grated or mashed

2 medium cloves garlic, grated or minced to a paste

1 to 4 Thai green chiles or serrano peppers, chopped

2 tablespoons chana masala spice blend

1 cup canned crushed tomatoes

1/2 teaspoon chaat masala spice blend, optional, for extra tang

Chopped fresh cilantro, for garnish

1 lime, cut into wedges

Instructions

Combine the chickpeas with the bay leaves, black tea bag, black cardamom, if using, 1 teaspoon salt and 2 cups of water in a large Dutch oven. Bring to a simmer over medium-high heat, then reduce to low and simmer until the chickpeas are soft and infused with the spices and tea, about 10 minutes. Discard the tea bag, bay leaves and cardamom pod. Drain the chickpeas and put them back in the pot they were cooking in.

Meanwhile, heat the ghee and/or oil in a large skillet or saucepan over medium-high heat. Add the onions and 1/2 teaspoon salt and cook, stirring and scraping occasionally, until the onions are very soft and golden brown, 10 to 12 minutes.

Add the ginger, garlic and green chiles and cook until the raw smell goes away, about 3 minutes. Add the chana masala along with 2 tablespoons of water and sauté until the raw smell dissipates, about 5 minutes. Add the tomatoes, 1/2 teaspoon salt and the chaat masala, if using, and cook until well cooked and pasty, about 8 minutes.

Add the spice mixture to the chickpeas with 1 cup of water, mix well and bring to a simmer over medium heat; simmer until the curry thickens, coats and infuses with the chickpeas, about 5 minutes. Adjust the salt to taste. Garnish with fresh cilantro and serve with lime wedges.

RECIPES FOR DINNER ON THE HASHIMOTO'S VEGETARIAN DIET

Sweet Potato Lasagna

Ingredients

Tomato Sauce:

3 tablespoons olive oil

1 small onion, diced

Kosher salt and freshly ground black pepper

2 cloves garlic, minced

One 28-ounce can whole peeled tomatoes

Lasagna:

Two 10-ounce boxes frozen chopped spinach, defrosted

1 pound mozzarella, grated

2 pounds ricotta cheese

1/2 cup grated Parmesan

1/4 teaspoon grated nutmeg

2 large eggs, lightly beaten

Kosher salt and freshly ground black pepper

3 pounds sweet potatoes (about 3 large)

Instructions

For the tomato sauce: Heat the oil in a medium saucepan over medium heat. Add the onions and 1/2 teaspoon salt and cook, stirring frequently, until softened and translucent, about 10 minutes. Add the garlic and cook for 2 minutes. Add the tomatoes and mash into a chunky puree using a potato masher. Bring to a simmer and partially cover the pan with a lid. Cook, stirring occasionally, until slightly thickened, about 30 minutes. Stir in 1/2 teaspoon salt and pepper to taste. Remove from the heat.

For the lasagna: While the sauce is cooking, drain the water from the spinach, place in a clean kitchen towel and wring well to remove any excess water. Break up the spinach into a large bowl. Set aside 1 cup of the mozzarella, then add the remaining mozzarella to the bowl with the spinach. Add the ricotta, Parmesan, nutmeg, eggs, 2 teaspoons salt and 1/2 teaspoon pepper and mix with a wooden spoon or rubber spatula until well combined.

Peel the sweet potatoes and trim a small bit from one of the longer ends on each so they will sit flat and not roll. Cut the potatoes lengthwise into 1/4-inch planks.

Preheat the oven to 350 degrees F.

To assemble the lasagna: Add about 3/4 cup of sauce to the bottom of a deep 9-by-13-inch baking dish. Place a single layer of sweet potato slices along the bottom. Top with one-quarter of the ricotta and spinach mixture and use an offset spatula or the back of a spoon to spread gently into an even layer. Dollop about 3/4 cup of sauce on top of the ricotta mixture. Top with another layer of sweet potato slices facing the opposite direction from the previous layer. Repeat with ricotta mixture and sauce until you have 4 layers, ending with the remaining sauce.

Cover the baking dish with foil and bake for 25 minutes. Remove the foil, top with the reserved mozzarella and bake until the lasagna is bubbling, the mozzarella is starting to brown and the sweet potatoes are tender when a paring knife is inserted into the center, an additional 45 to 60 minutes. Let sit for 20 minutes before slicing and serving.

Braised Chipotle Sweet Potatoes

Ingredients

1 teaspoon cumin seeds

1 tablespoon extra-virgin olive oil

2 large rainbow carrots, cut into 1-inch half-moons

1 large yellow onion, diced

2 large sweet potatoes (about 2 pounds), cut into 1-inch pieces

Kosher salt

6 cups kale (about 1 pound), woody ends discarded, leaves and stems chopped

Juice of 1 navel orange (about 1/3 cup)

1 tablespoon tomato paste

1 tablespoon dark brown sugar

1 chipotle pepper in adobo, seeded and chopped, plus 1 tablespoon adobo sauce, optional

1 1/2 cups vegetable broth

2 cups cooked brown rice, for serving, optional

2 radishes, cut into thin matchsticks

1/4 cup fresh cilantro, chopped

Instructions

Arrange an oven rack in the lower third of the oven and preheat to 350 degrees F.

Heat a large braiser or Dutch oven over medium heat. Add the cumin seeds and toast, stirring occasionally, until very fragrant, about 1 minute. Add the olive oil, carrots and onions and cook, stirring frequently, until the carrots soften and the onions start to become translucent, 3 to 4 minutes. Add the sweet potatoes and 1 teaspoon salt and toss together so that everything is coated with the oil and seeds. Cook until the sweet potatoes start to soften slightly on the edges, about 5 minutes.

Stir in the kale and 1 teaspoon salt and let wilt slightly, another 2 minutes. While the kale is cooking, stir the orange juice, tomato paste, brown sugar and chipotle into the vegetable broth. Add the adobo sauce, if using. Pour the mixture into the pot. Stir and toss all the vegetables with the broth mixture and bring the mixture to a boil. Taste for seasoning and add more salt if desired.

Cover with a lid and bake 30 minutes. Remove the lid, stir and bake, uncovered, until the potatoes are very tender and saucy, about 30 minutes more. Serve on a bed of brown rice if desired, topped with radish and cilantro.

Creamy Orzo with Mushrooms

Ingredients

8 ounces cremini mushrooms, thinly sliced

3 tablespoons extra-virgin olive oil

Kosher salt and freshly ground pepper

1 large leek (white and light green parts only), sliced and rinsed

2 cloves garlic, minced

12 ounces orzo

3 cups milk

1 1/2 cups shredded Italian cheese blend (about 6 ounces)

1 5-ounce package baby spinach (about 8 cups)

Grated zest and juice of 1 lemon

2 tablespoons chopped fresh parsley

Instructions

Preheat the oven to 425 degrees F. Toss the mushrooms with 2 tablespoons olive oil, a pinch of salt and a few grinds of pepper on a baking sheet.

Spread out in a single layer. Roast, stirring halfway through, until well browned and crisp around the edges, about 25 minutes. Let cool for a few minutes, then scrape up with a spatula and transfer to a bowl.

Meanwhile, heat the remaining 1 tablespoon olive oil in a large pot or Dutch oven over medium-high heat. Add the leek and garlic, season with salt and pepper and cook until the leek softens, about 2 minutes. Add the orzo, 2 cups water, the milk, 1 teaspoon salt and a few grinds of pepper. Bring to a boil, stirring constantly. Reduce the heat to a simmer and cook, stirring occasionally, until the orzo is al dente, 5 to 7 minutes.

Remove from the heat and add the cheese, spinach, lemon juice and 1 tablespoon parsley. Stir until the cheese melts and the spinach wilts; add a splash of water if the mixture is too thick. Season with salt and pepper.

Toss the mushrooms with the lemon zest and remaining 1 tablespoon parsley. Divide the orzo among bowls and top with the mushroom mixture.

Chickpea Stew

Ingredients

2 tablespoons plus 2 teaspoons Hungarian paprika

4 teaspoons ground ginger

2 teaspoons freshly ground black pepper

2 teaspoons ground turmeric

1/2 cup olive oil, plus more for serving

3 cloves garlic, chopped

1 large onion, chopped

Kosher salt

2 carrots, peeled and cut on the bias into 1-inch pieces

1 small poblano pepper, stemmed, seeded and chopped

One 14-ounce can diced tomatoes, preferably fire-roasted

2/3 cup Castelvetrano olives, pitted

Two 15-ounce cans chickpeas, drained and chickpea liquid reserved

1 small bunch curly kale, stemmed and torn into 3-inch pieces

Serving suggestions: labneh, chopped fresh parsley, Aleppo pepper, lemon wedges and toasted pita

Instructions

Mix the paprika, ginger, pepper and turmeric in a small bowl until combined; set aside.

Heat 1/4 cup of the oil in a large heavy pot or Dutch oven over medium-high heat. Add the garlic, onions and 1 tablespoon salt and cook, stirring and scraping occasionally, until the onions are very soft and golden brown, about 15 minutes. Add the carrots and poblano and cook until the colors brighten but the vegetables are not yet tender, about 3 minutes. Add half of the paprika mixture and stir to coat. Cook until the spices are very fragrant, 1 to 2 minutes. Add the tomatoes, olives, all of the chickpea liquid, half of the chickpeas and 1 cup water and bring to a boil. Reduce the heat to low, then cover and simmer until the vegetables are tender and the chickpeas are very soft, 35 to 45 minutes.

Meanwhile, position 2 oven racks in the upper and lower thirds of the oven and preheat to 400 degrees F.

Toss the kale, 2 teaspoons salt and the remaining 1/4 cup olive oil, chickpeas and paprika mixture in a large bowl until combined. Divide the kale mixture between 2 rimmed baking sheets and roast, tossing once, until the kale is charred in places, 15 to 25 minutes.

Serve the stew with the roasted kale and chickpeas and top with labneh, parsley, a sprinkle of Aleppo pepper, a squeeze of lemon and toasted pita.

Portobello Parmesan

Ingredients

1 tablespoon extra-virgin olive oil, plus more for the
dish

3 Portobello mushroom caps

1/4 teaspoon red pepper flakes

3 cloves garlic, smashed

1 28-ounce can diced tomatoes

4 fresh basil leaves

Kosher salt and freshly ground pepper

Kosher salt and freshly ground pepper

2 cups panko (Japanese breadcrumbs)

1 cup grated parmesan cheese

2 tablespoons chopped fresh parsley

4 large eggs

1 cup all-purpose flour

Peanut oil, for frying

4 ounces buffalo mozzarella cheese, sliced

Instructions

Preheat the oven to 350 degrees F. Lightly oil a 9-by-13-inch baking dish. Scrape out the gills of the Portobello's with a spoon, then halve the mushrooms horizontally to make 6 thin rounds.

Heat the olive oil in a saucepan over medium-high heat. Add the red pepper flakes and garlic; cook 1 minute. Reduce the heat to low, add the tomatoes and basil and cook until the garlic is soft, about 15 more minutes. Transfer to a food processor and puree until smooth. Season with salt and pepper.

Combine the panko, 1/2 cup parmesan, 1 tablespoon parsley, 1 teaspoon salt and 1/2 teaspoon pepper in a shallow bowl. Whisk the eggs and 2 tablespoons cold water in another bowl. Put the flour in a third bowl.

Dredge the mushrooms in flour, shaking off the excess. Dip in the eggs and then in the panko mixture, pressing to coat both sides. Heat 1/2 inch peanut oil in a large skillet over medium-high heat. Working in batches, fry the mushrooms until golden, about 2 minutes per side. Drain on paper towels.

Spread a layer of the tomato sauce in the prepared baking dish. Add the fried mushrooms, then cover with the remaining tomato sauce. Top with the mozzarella and the remaining 1/2 cup parmesan. Bake until browned, 20 to 25 minutes. Sprinkle with the remaining 1 tablespoon parsley.

Whole Roasted Cauliflower with Pomegranate and Tahini

Ingredients

Cauliflower:

One 2- to 2 1/2-pound head cauliflower

2 tablespoons olive oil

1/2 teaspoon ground cumin

1/2 teaspoon ground coriander

Kosher salt and freshly ground black pepper

1/4 cup loosely packed fresh parsley leaves

2 tablespoons toasted pine nuts

2 tablespoons pomegranate seeds

Flaky sea salt, such as Maldon, for garnish

Tahini Sauce:

1/4 cup tahini

1/4 cup lemon juice

2 tablespoons olive oil

1/4 teaspoon ground cumin

1 clove garlic, finely grated

Kosher salt and freshly ground black pepper

Instructions

For the cauliflower: Preheat the oven to 425 degrees F.

Remove the leaves from the cauliflower, then trim the stem flush with the bottom of the head so the cauliflower sits flat and upright. Transfer to a medium ovenproof skillet. Rub the outside of the cauliflower with the olive oil, then sprinkle evenly with the cumin, coriander, 1 teaspoon kosher salt and several grinds of pepper. Pour 1 cup water into the bottom of skillet, then wrap tightly with aluminum foil.

Bake until the cauliflower is crisp-tender, 40 to 45 minutes. Remove the foil and continue to bake until the cauliflower is very tender and golden brown, 30 minutes more. (The core of the cauliflower should be tender but the whole head should hold its shape and not fall apart.)

For the tahini sauce: Meanwhile, stir together the tahini, lemon juice, olive oil, cumin, garlic, 1/2 teaspoon kosher salt and several grinds of pepper until combined. Whisk in 3 to 4 tablespoons of water until the sauce is very smooth and creamy. The sauce may look lumpy at first, but will come together once the water is incorporated. Taste and adjust the seasoning with salt and pepper.

Transfer the cauliflower to a serving platter, then top with the parsley, pine nuts, pomegranate seeds and a pinch of flaky sea salt. Drizzle with some of the tahini sauce, then cut into wedges and serve with more tahini sauce on the side.

Charred Tomato Gazpacho

Ingredients

1/2 teaspoon cumin seeds

1/2 teaspoon coriander seeds, lightly crushed

1/2 cup plus 1 tablespoon extra-virgin olive oil

1/2 cup crustless white bread cubes

1 large clove garlic

Kosher salt

3 1/4 pounds tomatoes, halved

1/2 teaspoon sugar

2 tablespoons sherry vinegar

1 Kirby cucumber

1 green bell pepper

Freshly ground pepper

Instructions

Preheat a grill or grill pan to medium high. Heat the cumin seeds, coriander seeds and 1/2 cup olive oil in a small skillet over medium-low heat until the seeds are toasted, about 3 minutes. Transfer to a liquid measuring cup. Transfer 3 tablespoons of the spiced oil and about half of the seeds to a small bowl; reserve for topping.

Put the bread cubes in a bowl, cover with water and let soak 2 minutes. Drain, squeeze dry and set aside.

Mince the garlic, then sprinkle with a pinch of salt and mash it into a paste with the flat side of a knife.

Toss the tomatoes in a bowl with the remaining 1 tablespoon olive oil and grill until charred, about 3 minutes per side. Transfer half each of the charred tomatoes, bread, garlic paste, sugar and vinegar to a blender; add 1/4 teaspoon salt and puree until smooth. With the motor running, add about half of the spiced oil from the measuring cup. Pour the mixture through a fine-mesh sieve into a bowl. Blend the remaining tomatoes, bread, garlic paste, sugar and vinegar with the other half of the spiced oil and 1/4 teaspoon salt, then strain into the bowl. Chill the soup at least 2 hours.

Dice the cucumber and bell pepper. Season the soup with salt and pepper. Ladle into bowls; drizzle with the reserved spiced oil and top with the diced vegetables.

Frittata with Asparagus, Tomato and Fontina

Ingredients

6 large eggs

2 tablespoons whipping cream

1/2 teaspoon salt, plus a pinch

1/4 teaspoon freshly ground black pepper

1 tablespoon olive oil

1 tablespoon butter

12 ounces asparagus, trimmed, cut into 1/4 to 1/2-inch pieces

1 tomato, seeded, diced

Salt

3 ounces Fontina, diced

Instructions

Preheat the broiler. Whisk the eggs, cream, 1/2 teaspoon salt, and pepper in a medium bowl to blend. Set aside. Heat the oil and butter in a 9 1/2-inch-diameter nonstick ovenproof skillet over medium heat. Add the asparagus and sauté until crisp-tender, about 2 minutes. Raise the heat to medium-high. Add the tomato and a pinch of salt and sauté 2 minutes longer. Pour the egg mixture over the asparagus mixture and cook for a few minutes until the eggs start to set. Sprinkle with cheese. Reduce heat to medium-low and cook until the frittata is almost set but the top is still runny, about 2 minutes. Place the skillet under the broiler. Broil until the top is set and golden brown on top, about 5 minutes. Let the frittata stand 2 minutes. Using a rubber spatula, loosen the frittata from skillet and slide the frittata onto a plate.

Agnolotti with Artichoke Sauce

Ingredients

1 9-ounce package frozen artichoke hearts, thawed and coarsely chopped

1 cup half-and-half

1 clove garlic, smashed

1/8 teaspoon red pepper flakes

Kosher salt

1 cup frozen peas (do not thaw)

1 teaspoon finely grated lemon zest

2 teaspoons fresh lemon juice

1 pound refrigerated cheese agnolotti (moon-shaped stuffed pasta) or ravioli

1/4 cup finely grated parmesan cheese

1/4 cup torn fresh basil leaves

Instructions

Combine the artichokes, half-and-half, garlic, red pepper flakes and 1/4 teaspoon salt in a large skillet and bring to a simmer over medium heat. Cover and cook until the artichokes are tender, about 5 minutes. Add the peas and continue to cook, covered, until tender, about 5 more minutes. Remove from the heat and stir in the lemon zest and juice. Discard the garlic clove.

Meanwhile, bring a large pot of salted water to a boil. Add the agnolotti and cook as the label directs. Reserve 1/2 cup cooking water, then drain the pasta and transfer to the skillet with the sauce.

Add the parmesan to the skillet and gently stir until the pasta is coated. Thin the sauce with some of the reserved cooking water. Stir in the basil.

Vegetarian Skillet Chili Topped with Cornbread

Ingredients

Chili:

2 tablespoons vegetable oil

1 pound (about 4 cups) store-bought diced butternut squash, cut into 1/2-inch cubes

Kosher salt and freshly ground black pepper

3 cloves garlic, thinly sliced

1 medium onion, finely chopped

4 tablespoons chili powder, or to taste

2 teaspoons ground cumin

3 cups low-sodium vegetable stock

Two 14.5-ounce cans diced tomatoes with chiles, drained

One 14.5-ounce can kidney beans, drained and rinsed

1 tablespoons sugar

5 ounces (about 6 cups lightly packed) baby spinach

Cornbread Topping:

3/4 cup fine cornmeal

3/4 cup all-purpose flour

3/4 teaspoon baking soda

3 tablespoons sugar

Kosher salt

1/2 cup whole milk

1/4 cup sour cream, plus more for serving

1 large egg

3 tablespoons unsalted butter, melted

3/4 cup shredded Cheddar (about 3 ounces)

Pickled jalapenos, for serving

Instructions

For the chili: Heat the oil in a 12-inch cast-iron skillet over medium-high heat. Add the squash and a pinch of salt and black pepper and cook, stirring occasionally, until the squash is tender and browned in spots, about 8 minutes. Remove the squash from the pan and set aside.

Reduce the heat to medium. Add the garlic and onion and cook, stirring often, until the onion is soft, about 8 minutes. Add the chili powder (use less if you like milder chili) and cumin and cook until fragrant, about 1 minute. Add the vegetable stock, tomatoes, beans, sugar and cooked squash and bring to a simmer. Cook until all of the vegetables are tender and the sauce has thickened, about 30 minutes. (If the liquid reduces to less than three-quarters of the way up the sides of the squash, stir in a little water.) Stir in the baby spinach by the handful until all is incorporated and wilted.

For the cornbread topping: Meanwhile, position a rack in the center of the oven and preheat to 400 degrees F. Whisk the cornmeal, flour, baking soda, sugar and 1 teaspoon salt together in a medium bowl. Whisk the milk, sour cream and egg together in another bowl. Add the wet ingredients to the dry ingredients, whisking until well combined. Stir in the melted butter and Cheddar. Drop spoonfuls of the batter on top of the chili, leaving space in between. (The batter will not completely cover the chili.)

Bake until the cornbread is golden brown and springs back when touched and the chili is hot and bubbly, about 18 minutes. Serve with more sour cream and pickled jalapenos.

Beet Reuben

Ingredients

3 tablespoons mayonnaise

2 tablespoons chopped dill pickle

1 tablespoon ketchup

Dash of hot sauce

2 teaspoons ground coriander

2 teaspoons smoked paprika

1 teaspoon ground allspice

1 teaspoon ground mustard

Kosher salt and freshly ground black pepper

2 large cooked beets, peeled

4 slices rye bread

4 thick slices Swiss cheese

1 cup drained sauerkraut

2 tablespoons unsalted butter

Instructions

Mix the mayonnaise, pickle, ketchup and hot sauce in a small bowl. Mix the coriander, smoked paprika, allspice, mustard, 1/2 teaspoon salt and 1/2 teaspoon pepper in a shallow dish. Roll the beets in the spice mixture to coat. Slice the beets 1/4 inch thick.

Spread each slice of bread with the mayonnaise mixture. Lay 1 cheese slice on each of 2 slices of the bread. Top with the sauerkraut. Divide the sliced beets and arrange on top of the sauerkraut. Top with the remaining cheese. Close the sandwiches, mayonnaise-side down. Press lightly with your hand.

Heat a large skillet over medium-low heat. Add 1 tablespoon of the butter. When the butter is melted, add the sandwiches. Cook until golden on the underside, about 3 minutes. Add the remaining tablespoon butter, let melt, then flip the sandwiches. Cook until the underside is golden and the cheese is melted, about 3 minutes more. Cut the sandwiches in half before serving.

Mini Mac and 'Shrooms

Ingredients

Kosher salt

1 pound mezzi rigatoni

1 stick unsalted butter

1/2 cup all-purpose flour

4 cups whole milk

1/4 teaspoon freshly grated nutmeg

Freshly ground pepper

2 tablespoons extra-virgin olive oil

1 pound wild mushrooms, such as oyster or shiitake, stemmed and sliced

4 ounces cremini mushrooms, quartered

8 ounces taleggio or brie cheese, rind removed, cubed (about 1 1/2 cups)

5 ounces pecorino cheese, grated (about 1 1/2 cups)

1/2 cup breadcrumbs

2 tablespoons chopped fresh parsley

Instructions

Bring a large pot of salted water to a boil; add the pasta and cook until al dente, about 9 minutes. Drain the pasta, reserving about 1/4 cup cooking water.

Meanwhile, melt 4 tablespoons butter in a large skillet over medium heat. Stir in the flour with a wooden spoon to make a paste. Cook, stirring, until the paste puffs slightly, about 1 minute. Remove from the heat and gradually whisk in the milk until smooth. Bring to a boil over medium-high heat, whisking. Reduce the heat and simmer, whisking occasionally, until the sauce is creamy, 8 to 10 minutes. Add the nutmeg and season with salt and pepper.

Meanwhile, heat 2 tablespoons butter and the olive oil in a large skillet over medium-high heat. Add half of the mushrooms and cook until soft, about 8 minutes. Season with salt. Push to the side of the pan and repeat with the remaining mushrooms.

Reduce the heat under the sauce to low and whisk in both cheeses until smooth. Stir in the mushrooms and pasta and toss, adding the reserved cooking water as needed.

Melt the remaining 2 tablespoons butter in a skillet over medium heat. Add the breadcrumbs and toast until golden; stir in the parsley. Divide the pasta among 8 small bowls. Garnish with the breadcrumb mixture.

Chile Cheese Casserole

Ingredients

Nonstick cooking spray

4 cups baked tortilla chips, 2 1/2 ounces

6 egg whites

4 large eggs

1/4 cup skim milk

3/4 teaspoon ancho chili powder

1/8 teaspoon freshly ground black pepper

1 (4-ounce) can mild chopped green chiles

1 tablespoon chopped fresh cilantro leaves, plus whole leaves for garnish

1/2 cup shredded sharp Cheddar cheese, about 2 ounces

1/2 cup shredded pepper jack cheese, about 2 ounces

1/2 cup prepared green salsa verde

Reduced-fat sour cream, optional

Instructions

Preheat the oven to 375 degrees F. Lightly coat a rectangular 2-quart baking dish with nonstick cooking spray. Coarsely crush the chips by hand and spread half of them into the bottom of the baking dish.

Whisk the egg whites, eggs, milk, ancho powder, and pepper in a large bowl until well combined. Stir in the chopped chiles, chopped cilantro, and 1/4 cup each of the Cheddar and pepper jack cheeses; pour into the pan. Sprinkle the remaining chips over the egg mixture. Bake until the casserole is set around the edges but a little loose in the center, 20 to 25 minutes.

Sprinkle with the remaining 1/4 cup of each cheese and continue to bake until the cheeses are melted and the casserole is set in the center, about 10 minutes. Let stand 10 minutes. Serve with the salsa and, sour cream, if using. Garnish with whole cilantro leaves.

Vegetarian Pad Thai

Ingredients

Noodles:

5 ounces flat rice stick noodles (linguine size)

Sauce:

2 tablespoons packed brown sugar

2 tablespoons tamarind paste or tamarind concentrate

1 to 3 tablespoons sriracha (depending on desired heat level)

1 tablespoon lime juice

1 tablespoon low-sodium soy sauce

Stir Fry:

2 tablespoons vegetable oil

1 cup cubed extra-firm tofu (1-by-1/2-inch cubes)

1 shallot, thinly sliced

1 large egg, lightly beaten

1/2 red bell pepper, cut into thin strips

1 cup mung bean sprouts

3 thin scallions, cut diagonally into 1-inch pieces

1/4 cup roasted peanuts, chopped

1/4 cup fresh cilantro leaves

Lime wedges, for serving

Instructions

For the noodles: Cook the noodles according to the package instructions.

For the sauce: Stir together the brown sugar, tamarind, sriracha, lime juice and soy sauce in a small bowl until well combined.

For the stir fry: Heat the oil in a large nonstick skillet over medium heat. Add the tofu and shallots and cook, stirring occasionally, until lightly browned, 4 to 5 minutes. Push the tofu and shallots to the side, allowing the excess oil to drip down into the middle of the skillet.

Add the beaten egg to the middle of the skillet and cook, stirring occasionally and chopping to break it up, until cooked through, about 30 seconds. Add the peppers and cook just to soften slightly, about 2 minutes. Add the cooked noodles, bean sprouts, scallions and sauce to the skillet. Combine the tofu and egg into the ingredients and stir-fry, coating the ingredients with the sauce, and simmer to thicken, 3 to 5 minutes.

Pile the stir fry onto a serving plate and top with the peanuts and cilantro. Serve immediately with lime wedges.

Tofu-Vegetable Stir-Fry

Ingredients

1 cup white or jasmine rice

3 tablespoons low-sodium soy sauce

3 tablespoons hoisin sauce

2 tablespoons balsamic vinegar

1 tablespoon Asian chile sauce (such as Sriracha)

2 teaspoons cornstarch

2 tablespoons sesame oil

4 scallions, sliced (white and green parts separated)

2 cloves garlic, minced

1 1-inch piece ginger, peeled and finely chopped

4 ounces shiitake mushrooms, stemmed and chopped

4 ounces snow peas

1 14-ounce package soft tofu, drained and cut into 1-inch cubes

Instructions

Cook the rice as the label directs. Meanwhile, whisk the soy sauce, hoisin sauce, vinegar, chile sauce, cornstarch and 1 cup water in a small bowl until smooth; set aside.

Heat the sesame oil in a wok or large skillet over medium-high heat. Add the scallion whites, garlic and ginger and stir-fry 30 seconds. Add the mushrooms and stir-fry until golden brown and tender, about 3 minutes. Add the snow peas and stir-fry 30 more seconds.

Whisk the reserved soy sauce mixture and add it to the wok. Bring to a simmer, then add the tofu. Cook, stirring occasionally, until the sauce is thick, about 2 minutes. Sprinkle with the scallion greens.

Fluff the rice with a fork and divide among bowls. Top with the stir-fry and sauce.

RECIPES FOR SOUP ON THE HASHIMOTO'S VEGETARIAN DIET

Pasta e Ceci

Ingredients

3 tablespoons extra-virgin olive oil, plus more for drizzling

2 medium carrots, cut into 1/2-inch chunks

2 stalks celery, cut into 1/2-inch chunks

2 medium leeks, white and light green parts, halved lengthwise and sliced

3 tablespoons tomato paste

1 tablespoon fresh rosemary leaves, chopped

3 cloves garlic, chopped

Pinch crushed red pepper flakes

Two 15.5-ounce cans chickpeas, rinsed and drained

1 lemon, zest peeled in several long strips with a vegetable peeler, plus half of the lemon juiced

2 fresh bay leaves

1 Parmesan rind, about 3 inches long (optional), plus freshly grated Parmesan for serving

Kosher salt

1 1/2 cups ditalini

Instructions

Heat the olive oil in a medium Dutch oven over medium heat. When the oil is hot, add the carrots, celery and leeks; cook, stirring occasionally, until the leeks are wilted, about 5 minutes. Clear a space in the center of the pot and add the tomato paste, rosemary, garlic and red pepper flakes. Let toast for a minute, then stir into the vegetables. Add the chickpeas, lemon zest, bay leaves, Parmesan rind, if using, 6 cups water and 1 1/2 teaspoons salt. Bring to a simmer and cook, uncovered, until the vegetables are tender, 18 to 20 minutes. Use a potato masher to mash some of the chickpeas until the broth appears creamy and slightly thick, leaving plenty of chickpeas whole, 6 or 7 mashes around the pot should do the trick. Add the ditalini and 1 cup water. Return to a simmer and cook until the ditalini is very al dente, about 7 minutes. Remove from the heat, stir in the lemon juice and let sit until the broth is thickened and the pasta finishes cooking, about 5 minutes.

Remove the bay leaves, cheese rind and lemon zest before serving. Season the pasta e ceci with salt, if needed. Serve with a drizzle of olive oil and a sprinkle of freshly grated Parmesan.

Healthified Broccoli Cheddar Soup

Ingredients

1 bunch broccoli

1 small onion, finely chopped

1 medium red-skinned potato, diced

1/4 cup all-purpose flour

3 cups low-sodium chicken or vegetable broth

Kosher salt and freshly ground black pepper

1/4 teaspoon freshly grated nutmeg

1 cup grated extra-sharp Cheddar

1 teaspoon Worcestershire sauce

One 12-ounce can fat-free evaporated milk

2 scallions, thinly sliced

Instructions

Separate the stems and the florets from the broccoli. Trim and discard the bottom of the broccoli stems and peel the tough outer layers. Finely chop the stems and coarsely chop the florets and set aside separately.

Mist a large pot with nonstick cooking spray and heat over medium heat. Add the broccoli stems, onions and potatoes and cook, stirring, until softened, 7 to 10 minutes. Add the flour and cook, stirring, until lightly toasted, about 2 minutes. Stir in the broth and bring to a boil. Reduce the heat to maintain a simmer and continue to cook, stirring occasionally, until thickened and the vegetables are tender, 12 to 15 minutes.

Meanwhile, combine the reserved florets and 1/2 cup water in a small saucepan. Bring to a boil, cover and continue to steam until the florets are bright green and crisp-tender, about 5 minutes. Add the entire contents of the pot with the florets to the soup along with the nutmeg. Stir to combine and remove from the heat. Stir in the Cheddar, Worcestershire and milk. Season with salt and pepper. Garnish with the scallions.

Tomato Tortilla Soup

Ingredients

2 (6-inch) corn tortillas

1 tablespoon plus 1 teaspoon canola oil

1/4 teaspoon salt

1 small onion, chopped (about 1 cup)

3 cloves garlic, minced (about 1 tablespoon)

1 small jalapeno pepper, seeded and finely chopped

1 teaspoon ground cumin

3/4 teaspoon dried oregano

4 cups low-sodium chicken broth

2 (14.5-ounce) cans no salt added diced tomatoes with juice

1/4 cup fresh lime juice

1/4 cup reduced-fat sour cream

2 tablespoons chopped fresh cilantro leaves

Instructions

Preheat the oven to 375 degrees F.

Brush both sides of each tortilla with oil, using 1 tablespoon of the oil. Cut the tortillas in half, then cut each half into 1/4-inch wide strips. Arrange the strips on a baking sheet, sprinkle with the salt, and bake until crisp and golden, about 12 minutes. Remove from oven and set aside.

Heat the remaining 1 teaspoons of oil in a large heavy skillet over medium heat. Add the onion and cook for 5 minutes, stirring occasionally, until onion is soft and translucent. Add the garlic, jalapeno, cumin, and oregano and cook for 1 minute more. Add the broth and tomatoes, bring to a boil, then reduce the heat to low and simmer for about 10 minutes. Stir in lime juice.

Remove the pan from the heat and puree with an immersion blender or in 2 batches in a regular blender until the soup lightens in color but chunks of tomato remain, about 30 seconds. Serve the soup topped with the tortilla strips, a dollop of sour cream, and a sprinkle of cilantro.

Mushroom Hummus Soup

Ingredients

2 tablespoons extra-virgin olive oil

2 shallots, minced

1 1/4 pounds cremini mushrooms, sliced

Kosher salt and freshly ground pepper

2 cloves garlic, minced

2 tablespoons Madeira wine or brandy

6 cups low-sodium chicken broth

2 sprigs thyme

3/4 cup hummus

Grated zest and juice of 1 lemon

2 tablespoons roughly chopped fresh parsley

2 scallions, roughly chopped

Greek yogurt, for topping

Instructions

Heat the olive oil in a medium saucepan over medium-high heat. Add the shallots and cook until soft, about 3 minutes. Add the mushrooms, season with salt and pepper, and cook until the liquid from the mushrooms evaporates, about 15 minutes. Add the garlic and cook 1 minute. Add the Madeira wine and cook 2 minutes, scraping up any browned bits. Add the broth and thyme; simmer gently, stirring occasionally, about 30 minutes.

Discard the thyme sprigs. Stir the hummus into the soup. Transfer half of the soup to a blender and puree (remove the filler cap to let steam escape), then return to the saucepan and simmer 15 more minutes. Remove from the heat, stir in the lemon juice and season with salt and pepper. Mix the lemon zest, parsley and scallions in a small bowl. Ladle the soup into bowls and top with the yogurt and lemon-parsley mixture.

When blending hot liquid, first let it cool for five minutes or so, then transfer it to a blender, filling only halfway. Put the lid on, leaving one corner open. Cover the lid with a kitchen towel to catch splatters, and pulse until smooth.

Miso Soup

Ingredients

4 to 5 cups dashi, recipe follows

2 tablespoons brown miso paste, plus more to taste

2 tablespoons white miso paste, plus more to taste

6 ounces firm tofu, cut into 1/2-inch cubes

2 scallions, white and green, thinly sliced on the diagonal

2 tablespoons aji mirin (sweetened rice wine), optional

6 cups cold water

One 12-inch long piece of kombu, wiped with a damp cloth

One .88-ounce/25 grams package shaved dried bonito flakes

Instructions

In a saucepan heat the dashi and whisk in the miso pastes. Bring to a simmer and add the tofu, scallions, and mirin, if using. Remove from the heat and serve immediately.

In a saucepan, combine the water and kombu. Bring to a simmer, uncovered, over medium heat. Remove the kombu and discard. Bring the liquid to a boil, add the bonito flakes and immediately remove the pan from the heat. Allow the dashi to sit undisturbed for 2 minutes. Strain through a fine mesh strainer into a medium bowl. Discard the bonito flakes. Use immediately or store, covered, in the refrigerator for up to 3 days.

Healthy Dried Mushroom and Barley Soup

Ingredients

1 ounce dried porcini mushrooms (about 1 cup)

3 cups boiling water

2 tablespoons olive oil

2 medium carrots, finely diced

1 medium onion, diced

8 ounces cremini mushrooms, thinly sliced, optional

Kosher salt and freshly ground black pepper

4 cloves garlic, minced

2 tablespoons sherry vinegar

1 tablespoon tomato paste

1 tablespoon all-purpose flour

1/2 teaspoon dried thyme

1 cup pearl barley

4 cups low-sodium vegetable or mushroom broth

1/4 cup sour cream, for serving

Chopped fresh parsley, for serving

4 slices hearty white or sourdough bread, for serving

Instructions

Place the dried mushrooms in a medium bowl and cover with the boiling water. Let soak until well hydrated and softened, about 15 minutes. Strain through a fine-mesh sieve, reserving the liquid. Roughly chop the porcini and set aside.

Heat the olive oil in a large pot or Dutch oven over medium-high heat. Add the carrots, onion, cremini mushrooms if using, 1/4 teaspoon salt and several grinds of pepper. Cook, stirring occasionally, until all vegetables are tender and mushrooms are golden brown, 8 to 10 minutes.

Add the garlic, 1 tablespoon of the vinegar and the tomato paste to the pot, then continue to cook, scraping up any brown bits from the bottom of the pan with a wooden spoon. Sprinkle the flour and thyme evenly over the vegetables and cook, stirring, until flour is dissolved and no longer raw, about 1 minute. Stir in the barley, broth, reserved mushroom liquid and porcini, 1/2 teaspoon salt and several grinds of pepper. Bring to a boil, then reduce to a simmer, cover slightly and cook until the barley is tender and the soup has thickened and reduced slightly, 30 to 35 minutes.

Season with salt and pepper. Stir in the remaining 1 tablespoon vinegar and ladle into 4 bowls. Dollop with sour cream, sprinkle with parsley and serve with a slice of bread, for dipping.

Kale-Potato Soup with Bacon

Ingredients

3 slices bacon, chopped

1 3/4 pounds Yukon gold potatoes (about 3), peeled and diced

1 leek (white and light green parts only), halved lengthwise and thinly sliced

2 cloves garlic, minced

1 teaspoon chopped fresh rosemary and/or thyme

Kosher salt and freshly ground pepper

4 cups low-sodium chicken broth

1 medium bunch kale, stems removed, leaves chopped (about 10 cups)

1/4 teaspoon Worcestershire sauce

1 tablespoon extra-virgin olive oil

1 tablespoon sour cream

2 tablespoons chopped smoked almonds

Instructions

Cook the bacon in a large Dutch oven or pot over medium-high heat, stirring occasionally, until crisp, about 5 minutes. Remove with a slotted spoon and drain on paper towels.

Add the potatoes and leek to the drippings in the pot and cook, stirring, until the leek is slightly softened, about 3 minutes. Add the garlic, herbs, 1/4 teaspoon salt and a few grinds of pepper. Cook, stirring occasionally, until the vegetables are slightly browned, about 2 minutes. Add the chicken broth and 4 cups water and bring to a simmer; cover and cook 15 minutes. Add about three-quarters of the kale; continue cooking, covered, until wilted, about 5 minutes. Stir in the Worcestershire sauce.

Meanwhile, preheat the broiler. Toss the remaining kale with the olive oil on a baking sheet; season with salt and pepper. Broil until crisp, about 3 minutes.

Thin the sour cream with a splash of water. Working in 3 to 4 batches, puree the soup in a blender until smooth; reheat if needed. Serve topped with the sour cream, kale chips, bacon and almonds.

NOTE: When blending hot liquid, first let it cool for five minutes or so, then transfer it to a blender, filling only halfway. Put the lid on, leaving one corner open. Cover the lid with a kitchen towel to catch splatters, and pulse until smooth.

Spicy Bean Soup

Ingredients

3 tablespoons olive oil

2 onions, chopped

2 celery stalks, cut into 1/2-inch pieces

1 carrot, peeled and cut into 1/2-inch pieces

1 red bell pepper, cut into 1/2-inch pieces

6 cloves garlic, finely chopped

1/2 cup chili powder

1 tablespoon ground coriander

1 tablespoon ground cumin

2 teaspoons dried oregano

1 teaspoon dried crushed red pepper, optional

2 (14 1/2-ounce) cans diced tomatoes with juices

1 (11 1/2-ounce) can tomato juice

1 (6-ounce) can tomato paste

1 (3-inch) piece Parmesan cheese rind, optional

2 teaspoons salt, plus more to taste

8 cups vegetable or chicken broth

2 (15 1/2-ounce) cans garbanzo beans, drained and rinsed

2 (15-ounce) cans cannellini beans, drained and rinsed

1/2 cup dried green lentils

3 cups broccoli florets

2 zucchini, cut crosswise into 1/2-inch thick rounds

2 yellow crookneck squash, cut crosswise into 1/2-inch thick rounds

1/2 cup freshly shredded Parmesan

1/4 cup thinly sliced fresh basil leaves

Instructions

Heat the oil in a heavy large stockpot over medium-high heat. Add the onions, celery, carrot, bell pepper, and garlic, and sauté until the onions are translucent, about 15 minutes. Add the chili powder, coriander, cumin, oregano and crushed red pepper, and cook for 2 minutes. Stir in the tomatoes with their juices, tomato juice, tomato paste, cheese rind, and 2 teaspoons of salt. Add the broth, garbanzo beans, cannellini beans, and lentils. Stir in the broccoli, zucchini, and yellow squash. Bring to a simmer over high heat. Decrease the heat to medium. Simmer, uncovered, until the lentils are tender and the mixture thickens slightly, stirring often, about 20 minutes. Season the stew to taste with more salt, if desired.

Ladle the stew into bowls. Sprinkle with the shredded cheese and basil, and serve.

Hearty Italian Chicken and Vegetable Soup

Ingredients

1 tablespoon extra-virgin olive oil

1 onion, chopped

Pinch crushed red pepper flakes

6 whole sprigs, plus 1 tablespoon chopped flat-leaf
parsley

6 (3-inch) strips lemon zest, cut from 1 lemon

1 small head fennel, thinly sliced (2 cups), fennel
tops reserved

1 1/2 pounds bone-in chicken breasts, skin removed

8 cups low-sodium chicken broth

A 2-3 inch piece Parmesan rind, optional

2 carrots, sliced (1 cup)

2 stalks celery, sliced (1 cup)

Kosher salt

3 cups baby spinach

2 tablespoons grated Parmesan, plus extra for
passing

Lemon juice

Instructions

Heat the oil in a Dutch oven set over medium heat. Add the onion and crushed red pepper flakes and cook until the onions begin to soften, 5 minutes. Meanwhile, tie the parsley sprigs, lemon zest, and fennel tops together. Add the herb bundle, broth, 2 cups of water, and, if using, the cheese rind. Bring to a very gentle simmer and simmer until the chicken is just cooked through, about 8 minutes. Transfer the chicken to a cutting board and set aside until cool enough to handle. Remove the meat from the bones in large strips, and set aside.

Meanwhile, add the sliced fennel, carrots, and celery to the broth and season with salt, to taste. Continue to simmer until the vegetables are just tender, 5 minutes. Stir in the noodles and cook until just al dente, about 5 minutes. Stir in the reserved chicken, baby spinach, and Parmesan until the chicken is heated through and the spinach is wilted. Discard the herb bundle and cheese rind. Stir in lemon juice, to taste. Ladle the soup into serving bowls and serve with additional Parmesan for passing.

Minestrone with Parmigiano-Reggiano

Ingredients

3 tablespoons extra-virgin olive oil

1 large red onion, chopped

2 large stalks celery, chopped

4 cloves garlic, chopped

2 large carrots, diced

1/4 pound thinly sliced pancetta, cut into thin strips

1/2 head Savoy cabbage, finely sliced, blanched and drained

1/2 bunch Swiss chard, finely sliced

1 large waxy potato, cut into 1/2-inch cubes

4 cups low-sodium chicken stock

3 medium tomatoes, seeded and diced

1 bouquet garni (1 sprig rosemary, 4 sprigs thyme, 1 bay leaf and 1 bunch parsley, tied together with kitchen twine)

3 cups cannellini beans (canned or cooked dried beans)

1 cup spinach, coarsely chopped

Kosher salt and freshly ground pepper

Grated Parmigiano-Reggiano cheese, for topping

Instructions

231

Heat the olive oil in a 4-quart pot over medium-high heat. Add the onion, celery, garlic, carrots and pancetta and cook, stirring, until soft, about 5 minutes. Add 4 cups water, the cabbage, chard, potato, chicken stock, tomatoes and bouquet garni. Bring the soup to a gentle simmer and cook 25 to 30 minutes.

Place half of the beans (1 1/2 cups) in a food processor and process until smooth. Add the bean puree and the whole beans to the soup and simmer 10 minutes. Add the spinach and cook 2 more minutes. Season generously with salt and pepper. Ladle the soup into bowls and garnish with cheese.

Clam and Bacon Soup

Ingredients

1/2 cup dry vermouth or white wine

24 littleneck clams, scrubbed

1 tablespoon extra-virgin olive oil

3 slices bacon, chopped

1 head garlic, cloves roughly chopped

3 spring onions or scallions (white and light green parts only), thinly sliced

3 stalks celery, thinly sliced, plus chopped leaves for topping

Kosher salt and freshly ground pepper

1/3 cup all-purpose flour

1 cup fresh or frozen peas

1/2 cup half-and-half or light cream

1 small baguette, sliced

Instructions

Bring 4 cups water and the vermouth to a boil in a large pot over high heat. Add the clams, cover and cook until they start opening, 4 to 10 minutes; as the clams open, transfer them to a bowl using tongs. (Discard any unopened clams.) Strain the cooking liquid through a fine-mesh sieve into another bowl; set aside.

Meanwhile, heat the olive oil in a large saucepan over medium heat. Add the bacon and garlic. Cook, stirring occasionally, until the bacon starts to crisp, about 7 minutes. Add the spring onions, sliced celery, 1/2 teaspoon salt and a few grinds of pepper. Cook, stirring occasionally, until the vegetables soften, about 7 minutes.

Sprinkle the flour over the vegetables in the pan; cook, stirring, until incorporated, about 1 minute. Slowly add the reserved clam cooking liquid, stirring and scraping up any browned bits from the bottom of the pan. Bring to a simmer and cook until thickened, about 3 minutes. Season with salt and pepper.

Add the clams to the saucepan (remove from the shells and chop, if desired); add the peas. Cook until warmed through, about 2 minutes. Remove from the heat and stir in the half-and-half. Top with celery leaves and serve with the baguette.

Mushroom-Caraway Soup

Ingredients

2 tablespoons unsalted butter

1/4 teaspoon caraway seeds

10 ounces cremini or white mushrooms, thinly sliced

Kosher salt and freshly ground pepper

3 medium carrots, quartered lengthwise and cut into 1-inch pieces

4 cups low-sodium chicken broth

1 small red onion, finely diced

1 tablespoon red wine vinegar

4 slices pumpernickel bread

1/3 cup sour cream or creme fraeche

Instructions

Melt the butter in a saucepan over medium-low heat. Add the caraway seeds and cook until fragrant, about 1 minute. Add the mushrooms and cook, stirring, until they begin to wilt, about 5 minutes. Add 1/4 teaspoon salt, and pepper to taste. Add the carrots and broth, cover and bring to a simmer. Uncover and cook until the carrots are tender, 10 to 12 minutes. Season with salt and pepper.

Meanwhile, combine the onion, vinegar and a pinch of salt in a bowl and let marinate while the soup simmers. Toast the bread.

Divide the soup among bowls and top with sour cream and the marinated onion. Serve with the toast.

Fisherman's Stoup

Ingredients

Seafood Base

1 medium red onion, coarsely chopped

1 Fresno chile pepper, chopped

1 tablespoon fresh lemon zest

2 cloves garlic, grated

1/2 cup flat leaf parsley, a couple of handfuls

2 tablespoons fresh thyme leaves

2 fresh bay leaves

Fresh flat-leaf parsley

Soup base

1/4 cup extra-virgin olive oil

6 anchovy filets

4 small ribs celery, chopped

2 starchy potatoes, peeled and chopped into small dice

1 red pepper, cored and finely chopped

1/2 bottle lager beer (about 6 ounces)

1 (28-ounce) can diced tomatoes or chunky-style crushed tomatoes

2 cups chicken stock

1 pound cod, cut into chunks

1 pound sea scallops

1 loaf ciabatta or other crusty bread of choice, for serving

Instructions

For the seafood base:

Place the red onion, chile pepper, lemon zest, garlic, parsley, thyme, and bay leaves in a food processor and process ingredients into paste.

For the soup base:

In a Dutch oven, heat the extra-virgin olive oil and anchovies over medium-high heat, when the anchovies melt into the oil add the seafood base and stir 3 to 4 minutes then add the celery, potatoes, and red pepper and cover the pot 4 to 5 minutes to sweat them out, stirring occasionally. Deglaze the pot with beer. Add tomatoes and chicken stock and bring to a boil, simmer for 20 minutes or until it has reduced by a third, then turn off the heat, cool and store for a make-ahead meal.

To reheat: Reheat over medium-high heat. Crust up and warm bread in a hot oven. When the stoup comes to a boil, fold or nestle the cod and scallops into the liquid, and return to a bubble, cook for 5 to 6 minutes, until the fish is opaque and cooked through, then turn off the heat. Serve immediately with lots of bread for mopping.

Chickpea Soup with Spiced Pita Chips

Ingredients

1/4 cup extra-virgin olive oil

2 stalks celery, chopped

2 carrots, chopped

1 large onion, chopped

Kosher salt and freshly ground pepper

2 15-ounce cans chickpeas, drained and rinsed

1 15-ounce can diced fire-roasted tomatoes with green chiles

1 tablespoon ground cumin

1 1/2 teaspoons ground coriander

2 pocketless pitas

Juice of 1/2 lemon

Chopped fresh cilantro, for topping

Instructions

Preheat the oven to 375 degrees F. Heat 2 tablespoons olive oil in a large Dutch oven or pot over medium-high heat. Add the celery, carrots, onion, 1/2 teaspoon salt and a few grinds of pepper. Cook, stirring occasionally, until the vegetables are softened, 7 minutes.

Add 6 cups water, the chickpeas, tomatoes, 2 teaspoons cumin, 1 teaspoon coriander and 1/2 teaspoon salt. Bring to a simmer and cook, stirring occasionally and slightly mashing the chickpeas with the back of a spoon, until the soup thickens slightly, about 20 minutes. Season with salt and pepper.

Meanwhile, slice the pitas into thin wedges. Toss with the remaining 2 tablespoons olive oil, 1 teaspoon cumin, 1/2 teaspoon coriander and 1/2 teaspoon salt. Spread in a single layer on a baking sheet. Bake until golden and crisp, 8 to 10 minutes.

Stir the lemon juice into the soup just before serving. Top with cilantro and the pita chips.

3-Bean Minestrone

Ingredients

2 tablespoons extra-virgin olive oil, plus some for drizzling

1 1/8-inch-thick slice prosciutto di Parma, about 1/4 pound, optional

1 onion, chopped

2 to 3 ribs celery, finely chopped

2 carrots, peeled and finely chopped

4 cloves roasted garlic (from roasted tomato recipe), recipe follows

1 red chile pepper, finely chopped or thinly sliced (recommended: Fresno or Holland)

Salt and freshly ground black pepper

1 pound small potatoes, chopped or 1 cup small pasta

1 (15-ounce) can cannellini beans, drained

1 (15 to 15.5-ounce) can garbanzo beans, drained

5 ounces fresh, thin green beans, cut into thirds

1 small head escarole or small bundle chard, shredded

Lemon zest

Parmesan cheese, shredded, for topping

Hot, crusty bread for mopping

Parmigiano and Herb Fortified Stock

1 large rind trimmed from a hunk of Parmigiano-Reggiano cheese or a few small pieces rind perhaps saved-up

Herb bundle of several sprigs each fresh thyme, parsley and rosemary, tied

1 onion, peeled and quartered

2 ribs celery, sliced on angle

2 carrots, sliced on angle

Peeled rind of 1 lemon

2 fresh bay leaves

4 cups chicken stock

12 cups (3 quarts) water

Roasted Tomatoes

24 ripe organic vine tomatoes or large plum tomatoes

Several cloves garlic, crushed

Extra-virgin olive oil, for liberal drizzling

Instructions

Set aside or prepare the stock and roasted tomatoes.

Heat a large pot or Dutch oven over medium to medium-high heat, add extra-virgin olive oil, a couple of turns of the pan. Add the prosciutto and stir a couple of minutes. Add the chopped onions, celery, carrots, garlic, and chile pepper, season with salt, and pepper. If you are using potatoes, add them here. If you are using pasta, heat a second medium pot of water to a boil for the pasta and cook according to package instructions for al dente. Cool the pasta and drizzle with a touch of extra-virgin olive oil. Cover and store separately from the soup. Cover the pan and sweat the vegetables 10 minutes, stirring occasionally. Add the cannellini beans, garbanzo beans, prepared stock and prepared tomatoes. Bring the soup to a boil and add the green beans. Bring the soup back to a bubble, then turn off the heat and cool the soup. Store the soup in the refrigerator for a make-ahead meal.

To reheat the soup: Place the soup over medium-high heat. Crisp up the bread in a warm oven. When the soup comes to a boil, stir in the cooked pasta, escarole, and a little lemon zest. Turn off the heat when pasta is warmed through. Serve the soup in shallow bowls and top with cheese, a drizzle of extra-virgin olive oil, and crusty bread alongside for mopping.

Parmigiano and Herb Fortified Stock

For the stock:

Place the cheese rind, herb bundle, onion, celery, carrots, lemon rind, bay leaves, chicken stock, and water into a pot and bring to a bubble, then reduce the heat to a simmer. Simmer at least 1 hour, and then remove the rind, herb bundle, and vegetables with a slotted spoon or strainer.

Roasted Tomatoes

For the tomatoes:

Heat the oven to 500 degrees F.

Arrange the tomatoes on a baking sheet or baking sheets in a single layer. Scatter the garlic among the tomatoes, dress with extra-virgin olive oil to coat and season with salt and pepper. Roast the tomatoes until they burst and skins split and begin to char, about 30 minutes. Cool the tomatoes until cool enough to handle and peel. Place the tomatoes in a bowl.

PART 4: FINAL THOUGHTS

Hypothyroidism, characterized by an underactive thyroid gland, disrupts the body's metabolism regulation primarily governed by thyroid hormones like thyroxine (T4) and triiodothyronine (T3). This sluggish metabolism often leads to the storage of calories as fat, making weight loss challenging for individuals with hypothyroidism. However, metabolic rates vary among those with this condition due to factors such as body size, gender, age, activity level, and genetics.

Hashimoto's disease, a prevalent autoimmune disorder affecting mainly women, targets the thyroid gland, causing it to become underactive. This condition results in symptoms like weight gain, fatigue, hair loss, and constipation. Despite its challenges, understanding and managing Hashimoto's disease is possible with the right knowledge and support.

Hashimoto's disease, also known as Hashimoto's thyroiditis, stems from a complex interplay of genetic predisposition and environmental triggers. Although its exact cause remains unclear, a family history of autoimmune diseases and certain environmental factors like infections, toxins, and chronic stress are believed to contribute to its development.

Managing Hashimoto's thyroiditis involves adopting a nutrient-rich, whole-food diet to support thyroid function and alleviate symptoms. Regular physical activity, sufficient rest, and stress management techniques can further enhance well-being. Collaboration with healthcare professionals is essential to tailor a management plan suited to individual needs and promote overall health and symptom relief.